THE PRACTICE-BASED EDUCATOR

THE PRACTICE-BASED EDUCATOR

A Reflective Tool for CPD and Accreditation

By

VINETTE CROSS
ANN MOORE
JANE MORRIS
LYNNE CALADINE
ROS HILTON
HELEN BRISTOW

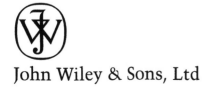

John Wiley & Sons, Ltd

Copyright © 2006   John Wiley & Sons Ltd
                    The Atrium, Southern Gate, Chichester,
                    West Sussex PO19 8SQ, England
                    Telephone (+44) 1243 779777

Email (for orders and customer service enquiries): cs-books@wiley.co.uk
Visit our Home Page on www.wiley.com

Other Wiley Editorial Offices

John Wiley & Sons Inc., 111 River Street, Hoboken, NJ 07030, USA

Jossey-Bass, 989 Market Street, San Francisco, CA 94103-1741, USA

Wiley-VCH Verlag GmbH, Boschstr. 12, D-69469 Weinheim, Germany

John Wiley & Sons Australia Ltd, 42 McDougall Street, Milton, Queensland 4064, Australia

John Wiley & Sons (Asia) Pte Ltd, 2 Clementi Loop #02-01, Jin Xing Distripark, Singapore 129809

John Wiley & Sons Canada Ltd, 6045 Freemont Blvd, Mississauga, ONT, L5R 4J3

Wiley also publishes its books in a variety of electronic formats. Some content that appears in print may not be available in electronic books.

Library of Congress Cataloging-in-Publication Data
The practice-based educator : a reflective tool for CPD and accreditation
    / by Vinette Cross . . . [et al.].
        p. ; cm.
    ISBN-13: 978-1-86156-422-1
    ISBN-10: 1-86156-422-8
    1. Medicine – Study and teaching (Continuing education) 2. Physicians – In-service training. I. Cross, Vinette.
    [DNLM: 1. Education, Continuing – methods. 2. Health Personnel – education.
3. Accreditation. W 18 P8958 2006]
    R845.P73 2006
    610′.7 – dc22
                                                                    2006001396

A catalogue record for this book is available from the British Library
ISBN-13 978-1-861-56422-1
ISBN-10 1-861-56422-8

Like guides, we walk at times ahead of our students, at times beside them, and at times we follow their lead. In sensing where to walk lies our art. For as we support [them] in their struggle, challenge them toward their best, and cast light on the path ahead, we do so in the name of our respect for their potential and our care for their growth. (L Daloz (1999) *Mentor: Guiding the journey of adult learners*, San Francisco: Jossey-Bass)

CONTENTS

CONTRIBUTORS

Vinette Cross PhD, MMedEd, MCSP, DipTP, CertEd
A physiotherapist by profession, Vinette has carried out doctoral research into undergraduate practice-based education and assessment. She has spent many years as a senior lecturer and researcher in pre- and post-registration education of physiotherapists, other allied health professionals and nurses. She has published in both professional and higher-education journals on clinical competence assessment, reflective practice and portfolio development. Vinette now divides her time between the roles of Visiting Senior Research Fellow in the Clinical Research Centre for the Health Professions at the University of Brighton and Senior Research Fellow in Ethnicity and Health in the School of Health, University of Wolverhampton. In addition, she advises on professional development and reflective practice as an independent consultant.

Ann Moore PhD, MCSP, DipTP, CertEd, MACP
Ann originally qualified as a physiotherapist and specialised in musculo-skeletal conditions. During her clinical years, she was a clinical educator for pre-registration students, and, after commencing an academic career at Coventry Polytechnic and later at the University of Brighton, she was involved in the preparation and support of clinical educators who were engaged in the delivery of undergraduate physiotherapy programmes. Ann led a team of authors in the development of *The Clinical Educator – Role Development* (1997), the predecessor of this current book. As a result, a postgraduate certificate in Clinical Education was developed at the University of Brighton. An active researcher since 1980, Ann has published over 80 peer-reviewed articles and is a regular keynote speaker at international and national conferences. She is committed to the development of practice-based educators as she sees this as crucial to the future of the allied health professions. Ann's current role is Director of the Clinical Research Centre for Health Professions at the University of Brighton. She is also Chairman of the National Council for Osteopathic Research and Chair of the Core Executive of the National Physiotherapy Research Network. She is a Fellow of the Chartered Society of Physiotherapy and a Fellow of the Manipulation Association of Chartered Physiotherapists.

Jane Morris MA, MCSP, PGCert (HE), ILTM

Jane is a Principal Lecturer and Clinical Education Tutor in the School of Health Professions at the University of Brighton. As clinical education tutor for two pre-registration courses and course leader for a Postgraduate Certificate in Clinical Education, she is actively involved in supporting student learning in practice settings and the role development of practice-based educators. Her research interests include facilitation of learning, collaborative models of practice education and interprofessional placement learning.

Lynne Caladine MSc, MCSP, DipTP, ILTM

Lynne is Head of the Division of Physiotherapy at the University of Brighton and Deputy Head of the School of Health Professions. After joining the university shortly after it opened in the early 1990s, Lynne was Clinical Education Tutor and subsequently Course Leader of the BSc (Hons) Physiotherapy course. Her extensive experience in professional education includes involvement in developing both a master's level module and a Postgraduate Certificate in Clinical Education at Brighton, and teaches on both. She is currently Chair of the Chartered Society of Physiotherapy steering group for the Accreditation of Clinical Educators (ACE).

Ros Hilton MSc, MCSP, DipTP, ILTM

Ros is Deputy Head and Senior Lecturer in the Academic Department of Physiotherapy, School of Biomedical and Health Sciences, King's College London, where she is currently Programme Leader for the BSc (Hons) in Physiotherapy. Most of her career has been spent in physiotherapy education, and in 1990 she gained a master's degree in the practice of higher education. Her teaching experience has spanned undergraduate and postgraduate learning. She has been involved also in developing and delivering continuing professional development courses for practice-based colleagues from the allied health professions and others, focusing in particular on educational role development and evidence-based practice skills. Her main interests are programme design and development, teaching psychological concepts with the potential to enhance physiotherapy practice, practice-based education and interprofessional learning in both university- and practice-based settings.

Helen Bristow MSc, MCSP

Helen is a physiotherapist with over 20 years' experience in a broad range of practice-related roles. This includes opening new placements in an underdeveloped service, working at regional level with practice-based education stakeholders to safeguard placements for courses that were running out and securing and opening up placements for new programmes. She also spent time on the Allied Health Professions Advisory Team at the Department of Health. Her experience of the broader political dimensions of healthcare and education in practice means Helen is well aware of the long-term positive impacts that high-quality practice placements can have on service quality and on staff recruitment and retention. For the last 10 years, Helen has been engaged in a range of project work in practice-based education for NHS trusts, higher education institutions and the Chartered Society of Physiotherapy, where she is currently Project Officer for the Accreditation of Clinical Educators (ACE).

FOREWORD

Continuing professional development must be part of the process of lifelong learning for all health care professionals – its purpose is to help professionals care for patients. (*Learning from Bristol – The Kennedy Report*, p. 340)

Allied health professionals practise in a constantly changing environment with patients, clients and carers as active partners in care. Allied health professionals are critical to delivering services that have a positive impact on those who use health and social care. They play an active role in influencing the development of future practice and services.

This book allows readers to explore their own learning and education as they develop skills to educate, support, mentor and influence the future development of professional practitioners; promoting innovation, new ideas and new thinking in the development of the next generation of professionals who will practise in different environments and organisations.

The quality of practice-based education is inextricably linked to the quality of service delivery. This text leads readers through current policy initiatives encouraging practitioners to continually reappraise the architecture of health and social care to identify new approaches and the implications for professional practice.

The text introduces readers to notable educators and thinkers who have researched and validated learning theories and explored adult learning pathways. This knowledge allows practitioners to appreciate the underlying concepts and philosophy of education whilst exploring their own development as self-directed learners. It will guide practice-based educators through the complexities of curriculum design and the educational approaches that underpin curricula. It will trigger an interest in further reading about the complexities of adult learning, helping practitioners to evaluate their own learning and formulate a personal orientation to education and professional practice. This will aid the development of readers as experts in clinical practice education and enable the development of skilled future practitioners who will enhance service delivery. It allows practitioners to develop a sound knowledge base to underpin clinical education as we move into a health and social care environment with evidence-based practice as the norm.

Allied health professionals are self-regulating professionals who recognise their own competence and learning needs: they have embraced equality and diversity and understand accountability and clear governance structures. This text will embed these essential components of good and safe practice challenging allied health professionals as learners to help students to address their own attitudes as they develop their learning and understanding of practice, its context and environment.

Above all this book will encourage practitioners to develop reflective skills, identifying their abilities as learners and practice-based educators, reasoners and practitioners facilitating self-awareness and personal growth. Those who use this text will be equipped with the skills to support change and transformation in patient care, developing their careers and realising their personal potential.

It is the assured, knowledgeable and reflective practitioner who will secure the future of allied health professionals; confident in their core purpose, competent to discharge their responsibilities, accountable for their actions and willing to challenge the status quo. It is these practitioners who will inspire, innovate and champion the interests of students, patients and the public.

Kay East
Chief Health Professions Officer
Department of Health

Kennedy I (2001) *Learning from Bristol. The report into the public inquiry into children's heart surgery at the Bristol Royal Infirmary 1984–1995.* CM5297(1) BRI.

PREFACE

The development of high-quality health professionals depends upon high-quality learning experiences in the practice environment. This is acknowledged by increased emphasis on quality assurance in practice-based professional education, and in calls for accreditation of practice-based educators. Inevitably, this has major benefits for patient/client populations utilising healthcare services.

This text builds on an earlier book, *The Clinical Educator – Role Development* (London, Churchill Livingstone), by Ann Moore, Ros Hilton, Jane Morris, Lynne Caladine and Helen Bristow. Published in 1997, it became a valued resource for practice-based educators in the allied health professions. For this updated version, Vinette Cross has joined the team. We hope this new book will prove equally effective in enriching the teaching and learning activities of practitioners in the practice setting. We did not set out to write a textbook per se; instead, we have created a practical learning text designed to enable practitioners to enhance their personal performance as practice-based educators.

The book uses a model of reflection to help practitioners develop confidence and self-efficacy in their ability to facilitate learning in the practice setting. Readers are led through each chapter by a series of exploratory reflective activities related to learning outcomes specified at the beginning of each chapter. These activities encourage readers to draw on their own practice experience and knowledge. At the end of each chapter pro formas are provided. These offer readers the opportunity to evidence their learning from each chapter, identify related learning needs and compile an action plan. In this way, the text contributes to portfolio building and acts as a resource for readers' continuing professional development.

We believe that enjoyable, fulfilling, high-quality practice-based learning experiences are crucial to ensuring a positive future for the allied health professions. We have written the book in a style we think is friendly and straightforward. We hope the experience of working through it will make a real contribution to enhancing learning experiences for practice-based educators and learners alike.

VC, AM, JM, LC, RH & HB

ACKNOWLEDGEMENTS

Our sincere thanks go to all those educators and learners, at every stage of professional development, whose insights, struggles and commitment to achieving quality in practice-based education provided the impetus and inspiration for this book.

1 ABOUT THIS BOOK AND HOW TO USE IT

Introduction For many years, the education of health professionals has involved a combination of institution-based learning in universities or colleges and practice-based learning within the clinical workplace. Increasingly, contributing to the education of learners in their particular areas of practice is an integral and recognised part of every health practitioner's professional role and responsibilities. We are all practice-based educators at some level or other, for example sharing in and supporting the learning experiences of our professional peers and colleagues, educating patients and carers or taking responsibility for planning and delivering award-bearing practice-based modules forming part of undergraduate or postgraduate programmes.

Who will find this book useful? We set out to write a practical text that provides an easily accessible resource for health professionals involved in practice-based education at a variety of levels. Therefore, this book has something to offer if you are:

- a practitioner for whom planning and facilitating practice-based learning are already core elements of your role as a health professional and you want to enhance your performance in that area;
- considering applying for formal professional accreditation as a practice-based educator;
- thinking about taking on a role in practice-based education but want to know more about what is involved;
- a practice-based learner yourself (e.g. on an undergraduate programme, an in-service junior rotation or a postgraduate practice-based module) who is keen to understand and contribute more effectively to the learning process.

What does the book aim to do? This book aims to provide a resource to help you learn about and understand the process of practice-based education and improve your skills as a practice-based educator. A key aim of the book is to help you think in detail about your role as an educator and develop it further through a process of reflection. In this chapter, we explain what that means by asking:

- What is reflection and what does it have to offer the practice-based educator?
- How can you organise your thinking to help improve your ability to reflect?
- How does this book use reflection to help you to develop your role?

We also suggest different ways to work through the book and explain how you could use the learning outcomes associated with each chapter to:

- build a portfolio of evidence of your learning and development as a practice-based educator for the purposes of continuing professional development (CPD) and professional re-registration;
- gain accreditation as a practice-based educator, if this is an opportunity offered by your professional body.

Learning outcomes Listed below are some learning outcomes associated with the aims of this chapter. Before continuing, consider how confident you feel now in relation to these learning outcomes and tick the appropriate box beside each one. Are there any personal learning outcomes you would like to add to the list?

	I am confident I can do this	I am not sure I can do this
1. Discuss the purposes of reflection in the practice setting.	☐	☐
2. Describe the components of a basic cycle of reflection.	☐	☐
3. Identify some different models of reflection.	☐	☐
4. List some performance outcomes relevant to accreditation or formal recognition as a practice-based educator.	☐	☐
5. Use this book as a resource to:		
o facilitate your personal development as a practice-based educator	☐	☐
o increase your capacity for effective action as a practice-based educator.	☐	☐

Think about any personal outcomes that you would like to add to this list and make a note of them.

> In order to benefit from accumulating experience, it is necessary to stop and think from time to time. (Roberts, 2002, p. 5)

What is reflection and what does it offer?

At its simplest, reflection is 'thinking' (Hewson *et al.*, 1989). For the purposes of this book, it means thinking about being a practice-based educator. Different definitions of reflection encompass different ideas about the purpose of this practice-oriented thinking, for example:

- identifying what you know or can do: thinking about what you do well as a practice-based educator and what areas need improvement – performance enhancement purposes;
- trying to discover and examine the assumptions and values that underlie what you do as a practice-based educator and trying to understand the reasons for your success or lack of it – self-awareness and personal growth purposes;
- confronting ethical dilemmas in your practice as an educator and becoming empowered to take action – ethical decision-making purposes.

Figure 1.1 shows that these purposes are not mutually exclusive. Areas of overlap exist, and individual acts of reflection will often encompass these overlaps – as we demonstrate later in this introduction.

Using the reflective process to fulfil these purposes can help you to:

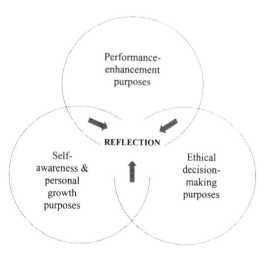

Figure 1.1. Overlapping purposes for reflection.

- stand outside your practice and see what you do from a wider perspective (Brookfield, 1998);
- make rational choices and be accountable for your own actions and decisions as a practice-based educator (Korthagen & Wubbels, 1995);
- use your own experience as an educator effectively as a resource for your own learning and CPD (Hewson, 1991).

How is reflective thinking organised?

Much has been written about 'how to reflect'. A basic and often used cycle of reflection, described by Kolb (1984), involves four stages, and these usually appear in some shape or form in models of reflection described by other writers. They are illustrated in Figure 1.2; we have used our own words to describe what is happening at each stage.

Stage 1. Thinking about and/or describing to someone else some aspect of your own experience;

Stage 2. Asking yourself some critical questions about your thoughts, feelings and actions (Johns, 1998; Gibbs, 1988) and/or being questioned by someone else, for example:
What were you thinking and feeling?
What was I trying to achieve?
What else could you have done?
How did my actions match my beliefs?
Why did I respond as I did?

Stage 3. Considering how learning gained from that particular experience could influence your practice in other areas (generalising);

Stage 4. Testing out improvements or changes based on your learning from the experience (experiential learning).

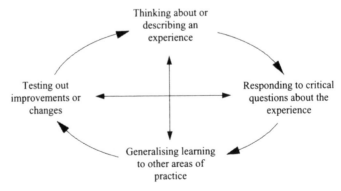

Figure 1.2. A basic cycle of reflection (adapted from Kolb, 1984).

Depending on what is appropriate or most useful in relation to a particular aspect of experience, you might reflect all the way round the cycle or you might choose to cut across it at various points, as shown in Figure 1.2.

How can reflection help to make sense of experience?

Figure 1.3 shows an example, unrelated to practice, of how elements of an experience might be fitted around a reflective framework. Firstly, elements of the experience are described in a factual way. Secondly, questioning reveals an ethical dilemma at the heart of the experience, and the assumptions and values underlying the action. Thirdly, the experience stimulates new insights into other behaviour and suggests how

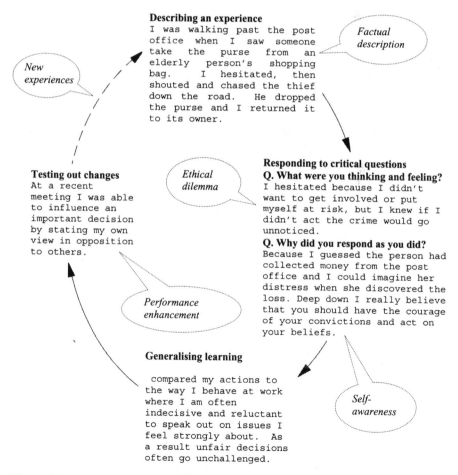

Describing an experience
I was walking past the post office when I saw someone take the purse from an elderly person's shopping bag. I hesitated, then shouted and chased the thief down the road. He dropped the purse and I returned it to its owner.

Factual description

New experiences

Testing out changes
At a recent meeting I was able to influence an important decision by stating my own view in opposition to others.

Ethical dilemma

Responding to critical questions
Q. What were you thinking and feeling?
I hesitated because I didn't want to get involved or put myself at risk, but I knew if I didn't act the crime would go unnoticed.
Q. Why did you respond as you did?
Because I guessed the person had collected money from the post office and I could imagine her distress when she discovered the loss. Deep down I really believe that you should have the courage of your convictions and act on your beliefs.

Performance enhancement

Generalising learning

compared my actions to the way I behave at work where I am often indecisive and reluctant to speak out on issues I feel strongly about. As a result unfair decisions often go unchallenged.

Self-awareness

Figure 1.3. An example of reflective thinking.

performance in other areas could be enhanced. Finally, this is tested out when an opportunity occurs. The way is then open for a new cycle to be initiated.

> [Reflection is] a generic term for those intellectual and effective activities in which individuals engage to explore their experiences in order to lead to a new understanding and appreciation. (Boud *et al.*, 1985, p. 19)

In this example, thinking critically about an experience in one context (acting with conviction in accordance with personal beliefs) raises echoes of previous experience in another context (when actions did not match beliefs). Examining the previous experience in light of new learning or insights (a process known as 'reframing') can lead to new ways of acting or responding when similar situations arise again.

How does the book use reflection to help develop your role?

Each chapter in the book provides you with opportunities to reflect or, in other words, to 'stop and think'. But, as Boud *et al.* (1985) emphasise, reflection is not *only* about thinking. It involves action, both as part of the reflective process and in response to it. At the start of each chapter, we ask you to engage in some preparatory reflection to help open your mind to what follows and enable you to think about your needs and goals in relation to the chapter's learning outcomes. In terms of reading the chapter, think of this as *preparing for action* (Cowan, 1998). Throughout each chapter, we introduce a variety of exploratory reflective activities to help you explore the concepts and issues raised in the text in relation to your own practice context. This often involves you in reframing previous experiences. Reflection is not an isolated activity; so many of the activities encourage you to engage in discussion with others, for example colleagues, mentors or critical friends. In terms of reading the chapter, think of this as *reflecting in action* (Schon, 1987).

After working your way through each chapter, we ask you to produce a piece of reflective evidence of your learning from the chapter for your professional portfolio. We also ask you to think about how you will take your learning forward into your future practice as an educator. In terms of reading the chapter, think of this as *reflecting on action* (Schon, 1987).

In Figure 1.4, Cowan's (1998) looped model of reflection has been adapted to illustrate how these 'stop and think' points in each chapter fit together. Within each loop, you may find yourself reflecting at one or more stages in Kolb's reflective cycle.

At the end of each chapter, we use this symbol to prompt you to think about and discuss with others the different ways the chapter has helped you to reflect upon

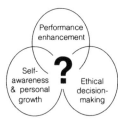

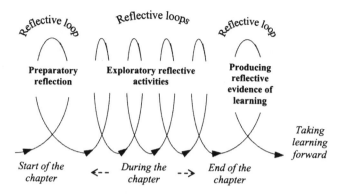

Figure 1.4. Process of reflection through each chapter using Cowan's looped model (adapted from Cowan, 1998).

a particular issue or aspect of your role as a practice-based educator. In other words, what purpose(s) did the chapter serve for you?

How can the book help to provide evidence for CPD?

CPD is learning that develops practitioners' knowledge and skills beyond the minimum required to register (Health Professions Council, 2004). It involves a wide range of learning experiences and is shaped by the individual's scope of practice and professional role. Providing evidence of CPD is the way in which regulatory bodies such as the Health Professions Council, General Optical Council, Nursing and Midwifery Council, General Medical Council, General Osteopathic Council etc. ask healthcare professionals to satisfy their registration requirements. This means being able to explain clearly:

- what you have learned over a particular period and what you can do;
- how you are applying the learning within your practice;
- what you are able to achieve in practice as a result.

Using learning outcomes

As you will have seen, each chapter starts with a list of learning outcomes. These provide a focus for your own assessment of how far working through the concepts and activities included in the chapter has helped increase your capacity for effective action as a practice-based educator. If, as suggested, you decide to add some learning outcomes of your own to the list, make sure they are achievable and not too difficult to assess. (Chapter 6 contains more information on how to write learning outcomes.)

Glossary   Words are the tools of reflective practice and CPD. Therefore, an important purpose of this book is to increase your confidence in putting your experience and expertise into appropriate language, which demonstrates clearly to regulators and other stakeholders your value and effectiveness as a practice-based educator. Every area of professional practice has its own specialist jargon, which can be confusing for the newcomer. Practice-based education is no exception. Therefore, a glossary is provided at the end of the book to help readers who are new to the area to build their vocabulary where necessary and gain confidence in using the specialist language and terminology of practice-based education.

Guided reading   To help you in compiling an evidence base for your practice as an educator, at various points in each chapter we suggest you read a relevant article that expands on some of the concepts introduced in the text. In addition, every chapter contains a bibliography of books and articles cited directly in the chapter itself, as well as some suggestions for further reading. A few texts in both lists are marked with asterisks to help you make a start on selecting reading appropriate for your particular needs and level of experience:

** Suitable for readers who wish to examine concepts at a more detailed or advanced level.
* Suitable for readers looking for something to stimulate ideas in a straightforward way.

Portfolio materials   At the end of each chapter (including this one), we provide a portfolio sheet that you could use in performance appraisal or CPD monitoring. This is based on your application of reflective activities in the chapter to your own practice as an educator and linked to your achievement of the chapter's learning outcomes. In Chapter 2, there is space on the sheet for you to consider your readiness to seek accreditation and/or other formal recognition as a practice-based educator, where this is appropriate. From Chapter 3 onwards, you can link evidence of your educator role to a set of outcomes for accreditation, which are listed in Box 1.1. The sheets also include an action plan for developing your learning further.

Working through the book   Each chapter in the book builds on learning acquired in earlier chapters. Where a chapter introduces a lot of new concepts or information, we make suggestions about how you might approach it. Frequent opportunities are

> **Box 1.1. Accreditation outcomes for practice-based educators**
> (adapted from CSP, 2004)
>
> 1. Describe the role and identify the attributes of the effective clinical educator. (Chapter 3)
> 2. Establish an optimal environment for effective learning. (Chapter 4)
> 3. Apply learning theories that are appropriate for adult and professional learners. (Chapter 5)
> 4. Plan, implement and facilitate learning in the clinical setting. (Chapter 6)
> 5. Apply sound principles and judgement in the assessment of performance in the clinical setting. (Chapter 7)
> 6. Evaluate the learning experience. (Chapter 8)
> 7. Reflect on experience and formulate action plans to improve future practice. (Chapter 9)

provided to work back and forth between chapters to revise and consolidate your knowledge and skills. Chapter 9 is designed to help you gain a clear picture of what you have learnt and achieved as a result of working through the book.

Summary

> This chapter has explained the rationale and aims of this book. Important points to consider are:
>
> - The book is intended as a flexible learning resource for allied health professionals interested in or actively involved with practice-based education at a variety of levels.
> - Reflection is a practical way to organise learning and thinking about your role and expertise as a practice-based educator.
> - A wide range of activities is provided to cater for individual and group reflection and learning about the practice-based education process.
> - Involvement in practice-based education provides a rich source of evidence of continuing professional development.
> - The book provides a format for collating evidence suitable for accreditation as a practice-based educator, in addition to wider professional-development purposes.

Now complete the portfolio sheet for Chapter 1.

- Respond to each of the questions regarding your feelings about being a practice-based educator.
- Reassess your confidence in relation to Chapter 1's learning outcomes listed on p. 2, including any personal learning outcomes you identified for yourself.

- Identify your development needs.
- Complete your action plan.

Finally, consider the different ways in which Chapter 1 has helped you think about your role as a practice-based assessor. What reflective purposes has the chapter served for you?

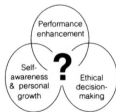

Portfolio Sheet – Introduction

Think about the questions below and record your thoughts in the space provided. You will have an opportunity to revisit your initial thoughts at the end of the book.

Q1. What is the point of being a practice-based educator?

Q2. What does it involve?

Q3. How do I see my role as a practice-based educator?

Q4. What activities do I engage in as a practice-based educator?

Q5. What qualities do I bring to my role as a practice-based educator?

Q6. What challenges do I face?

Q7. What rewards are there for me as a practice-based educator?

DEVELOPMENT NEEDS

ACTION PLAN

Chapter 1's Learning Outcomes

	I am confident I can do this	I am not sure I can do this
1. Discuss the purpose of reflection in the practice setting.	☐	☐
2. Describe the components of a basic cycle of reflection.	☐	☐
3. Identify some different models of reflection.	☐	☐
4. List some performance outcomes relevant to accreditation or formal recognition as a practice-based educator.	☐	☐
5. Use this book as a resource to:	☐	☐
o facilitate your personal development as a practice-based educator	☐	☐
o increase your capacity for effective action as a practice-based educator.	☐	☐
Personal learning outcomes for Chapter 1	☐	☐

Bibliography

Boud D, Keough R, Walker D (1985) *Reflection: Turning Experience into Learning.* London: Kogan Page.

*Brookfield S (1998) Critically reflective practice. *The Journal of Continuing Education in the Health Professions*, 18, 197–205.

Chartered Society of Physiotherapy (2004) *Accreditation of Clinical Educators (ACE).* London: CSP.

**Cowan J (1998) *On Becoming an Innovative University Teacher: Reflection in Action.* Buckingham: The Society for Research into Higher Education & Open University Press.

Gibbs G (1988) *Learning by Doing: A Guide to Teaching and Learning Methods.* Oxford: Further Education Unit Oxford Polytechnic.

Health Professions Council (2004) Consultation on CPD <http://www.hpc-uk.org/consultation.cpd.htm> (accessed 5 August 2005).

Hewson MG (1991) Reflection in clinical teaching: an analysis of reflection-on-action and its implications for staffing residents. *Medical Teacher*, 13(3), 227–231.

Hewson MG, Jensen NM, Hewson PW (1989) Reflection in residency training in the general internal medicine clinic. Paper presented at the annual meeting of the American Educational Research Association, San Francisco, CA.

Johns C (1998) Opening the doors of perception. In Johns C, Freshwater D (eds), *Transforming Nursing Through Reflective Practice*, Chapter 6. London: Blackwell Science.

Kolb DA (1984) *Experiential Learning.* Englewood Cliffs, NJ: Prentice-Hall.

Korthagen FAJ, Wubbels T (1995) Characteristics of reflective practitioners: towards an operationalisation of the concept of reflection. *Teachers and Teaching: theory and practice*, 1(1), 51–71.

*Roberts AE (2002) Advancing practice through continuing professional education: the case for reflection. *British Journal of Occupational Therapy*, 65(5), 2–6.

Schon DA (1987) *Educating the Reflective Practitioner.* San Francisco: Jossey Bass.

Further reading

Boud D, Docherty P, Cressey P (eds) (2005) *Productive Reflection at Work.* London: Routledge.

*Cross V (1993) Introducing physiotherapy students to the idea of 'reflective practice'. *Medical Teacher*, 15(4), 293–307.

Cross V, Liles C, Conduit J, Price J (2004) Linking reflective practice to evidence of competence: a workshop for allied health professionals. *Reflective Practice*, 5(1), 3–31.

*Ghaye, T, Cuthbert S, Danai K, Dennis D (1996) *Learning Through Critically Reflective Practice: Self-supported Learning Experiences for Health Care Professionals.* Newcastle upon Tyne: Pentaxion Limited.

Kinsella EA (2000) *Professional Development and Reflective Practice: Strategies for Learning Through Professional Experience.* Ottawa, Ontario: CAOT Publications ACE.

**Leitch R, Day C (2001) Reflective processes in action: mapping personal and professional contexts for learning and change. *Journal of In-Service Education*, 27(2), 237–259.

** Suitable for readers who wish to examine concepts at a more detailed or advanced level.
* Suitable for readers looking for something to stimulate ideas in a straightforward way.

2 PRACTICE-BASED LEARNING AND HEALTHCARE QUALITY

Introduction   The future of any healthcare profession is largely dependent upon the quality of the learning opportunities it provides for future generations of practitioners as they work towards professional registration, and also for its qualified membership as they continue to enhance and develop their professional knowledge and skills. Practice-based educators are key players in this process of assuring the future for their respective professions.

Historically, mechanisms for assuring and enhancing the quality of practice-based learning in the UK have focused on components delivered in higher-education institutions (HEIs) such as universities or colleges. Little scrutiny of practice-based elements has occurred. More recently, establishing a shared and efficient quality-assurance framework that engages service providers and practitioners in more equal partnership with higher-education providers has become a political priority. In this chapter, we review some of the significant features of this partnership. We begin by considering the changing nature of practice-based learning and the broadening role of practice-based educators. Later in the chapter, we review a selection of documents that illustrate the influence of wider health and education policy on practice-based learning. We also take the opportunity to clarify some of the terminology used to describe the process of practice-based learning.

- Depending on your immediate interests, you could read this chapter in full, or decide to come back to the documents later and consider their impact in relation to specific issues, as you work through the book.
- However, in Chapter 1 we suggested you use the portfolio sheets at the end of each chapter to gather evidence of your development as a practice-based

educator. Therefore, you might want to take particular note of the reflective exercise related to accreditation of practice-based educators on p. 29.

PREPARATORY REFLECTION Working through this chapter should enable you to achieve the learning outcomes listed below. Before continuing, consider how confident you feel now in relation to these outcomes and tick the appropriate box beside each one. Are there any personal learning outcomes you would like to add to this list?

Learning outcomes

	I am confident I can do this	I am not sure I can do this
1. Discuss the range of learning that takes place in your own practice context.	☐	☐
2. Identify key stages in the evolution of practice-based education in your own profession.	☐	☐
3. Identify terminology and models related to practice-based learning used in your own and other health professions with whom you work and collaborate.	☐	☐
4. Explain the reasons for the growing importance of practice-based learning and practice-based educators in terms of healthcare quality.	☐	☐
5. Discuss existing factors that influence further development of practice-based learning and the practice-based educator's role.	☐	☐

Think about any personal outcomes that you would like to add to this list and make a note of them.

What is practice-based learning?

The most essential and wide-ranging element of learning in the health professions takes place in the workplace, in other words, the practice setting. As notions of what constitutes practice-based learning expand, so the diversity of levels and modes of learning undertaken by practitioners in the workplace has increased. The idea of practice-based learning is associated automatically with traditional undergraduate, pre-registration programmes in which practice placements are a focus for the integration of campus-based and practice-based learning. But, as Figure 2.1 illustrates, it is increasingly associated with other types or levels of modules and programmes, for example:

- graduates on accelerated master's degree (MSc) qualifying programmes;
- practitioners taking postgraduate specialist practice MSc modules;
- assistant staff working towards vocational qualifications or foundation degrees;
- practitioners engaged in practice-based doctoral (PhD) research.

We must also recognise that experiential work-based learning provides the most effective means for practitioners to acquire specific and changing knowledge and skills required to continue practising effectively in healthcare organisations. In this context, many practitioners are now seeking transferable credit, or recognition of learning, by evidencing their experiential learning through portfolio development.

> ... learning is structured by the everyday activities and goals of the workplace. Given that these activities are necessarily important to the workplace, these learning experiences, and their outcomes cannot be considered to be incidental, ad hoc or informal. Rather, they are authentic and rich opportunities to reinforce and extend individuals' knowledge. (Billet, 1999, pp. 151–152)

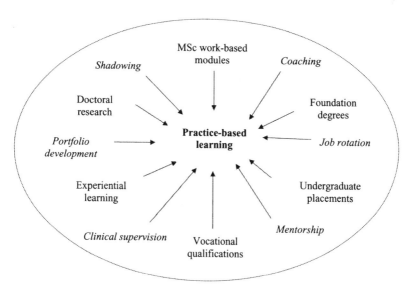

Figure 2.1. Diverse aspects of practice-based learning.

Mechanisms to facilitate this range of practice-based learning include mentoring, coaching, job rotation and shadowing, and non-hierarchical clinical supervision.

The terminology used for these practice experiences varies between (and sometimes within) professions and has evolved over time in each. Terms such as 'practice-based placement', 'fieldwork placement' and 'in-service block' are in common use. The precise pattern, duration and emphasis of placements are also subject to much variation. However, all must contribute to quality by ensuring learners at any level of experience are:

- fit for academic award (where appropriate);
- fit for practice and hence eligible for membership of the relevant professional body and statutory registration;
- fit for purpose in so far as they meet the immediate needs of employers and the service.

EXPLORATORY REFLECTION 2.1

- Talk to a range of colleagues and identify the variety of levels and types of learning currently occurring in your own workplace.
- How is this learning being facilitated and by whom?

Practice-based educators   Traditionally, practice–based educators are experienced work-based practitioners with a high level of knowledge and skill in a specialist field who accept responsibility for specific parts of the professional learning experience. In addition to an educational role with particular learners, they may be responsible for clinical units and personal caseloads. Their activities may involve education of pre-registration learners, newly qualified and novice learners within their own discipline, as well as more experienced practitioners and learners from other health professions. However, as the concept of team working becomes more established and sophisticated, practitioners of all grades are adopting an educative role in a variety of learning relationships with peers and colleagues within and across disciplines, for example by contributing to in-service education programmes or involvement in action learning sets. Although these activities may not involve a formal role as 'practice-based educator', all practitioners seeking to make a more effective contribution to learning in their own practice environment will find principles and ideas included in this book that can help them enhance the quality of learning experiences and outcomes. This includes allied health professionals in consultant roles who may be responsible for building an educational and learning culture in their practice environments.

Terminology: The title used for practice-based educators varies between and to some extent within professions. The terms 'practice-based educator', 'fieldwork educator', 'mentor' and 'practice-based supervisor' can all indicate a similar role. In the case of pre-registration learners, responsibility for practice-based learning is shared with campus-based educators at the university. These may be clinical-education tutors, who provide organisational and supportive liaison for practice-based educators and learners or they may be specific visiting tutors, who spend time with learners and educators in the workplace.

EXPLORATORY REFLECTION 2.2

In most health professions, there have been gradual but significant changes over the last few decades in the nature of practice-based placements and in the precise role of the practice-based educator.

Talk to a sample of senior members of your profession about their experiences as learners in the practice setting. Suggestions for questions you might ask are:

- How was your practice placement experience structured?
- What role did your practice-based educator play?
- How much support or help did you receive?
- How would you sum up the changes that have occurred in practice-based learning over the years?

You will probably find as we did that if you ask a representative sample of experienced practitioners the consensus will be:

- more structure now;
- greater support now, educators take more responsibility;
- more emphasis on meeting learners' needs now and less on providing 'an extra pair of hands';
- changing role of the practitioner in relation to learners – from passive overseer or supervisor to a more active participant in the learning process (Cross, 1994).

The role of practice-based educator is increasingly valued and rewarded. However, its effective fulfilment still presents a challenge for practitioners, and obstacles to its development still exist within the health professions. Figure 2.2 uses a force-field analysis (Lewin, 1951) to illustrate the forces driving the development of practice learning and the practice-educator's role and those forces that still exercise a restraining influence on attempts to move forward.

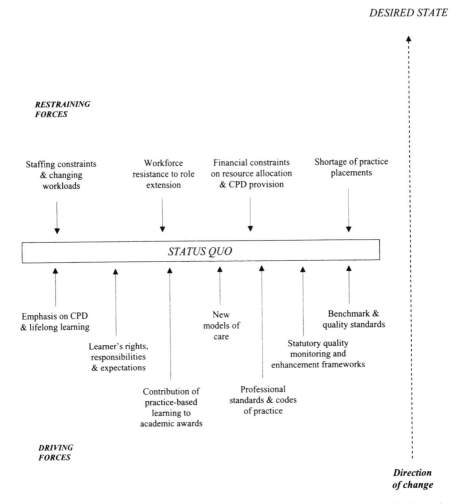

Figure 2.2. Analysis of the forces influencing the development of practice learning and the practice-based educator's role.

EXPLORATORY REFLECTION 2.3

- Discuss the force-field analysis with a group of colleagues. Are you aware of any recent policies, papers or initiatives that you want to add as either driving or restraining influences?
- Can you suggest any ways in which the power of the forces in either direction might be increased or modified?

The scope of the practice-based educator's role

At the start of the chapter, we commented on the broad scope of the practice-based educator's role. Below are some examples of ways in which practitioners can be involved in facilitating practice-based learning.

- A senior occupational therapist in a social services setting has two novice practitioners on rotation for a six-month period. As qualified staff, they work autonomously, but the senior facilitates their continuing professional development (CPD).
- A paramedic who is a specialist in resuscitation techniques provides in-service training for a range of other health professionals in order to ensure staff are adequately prepared to use life-saving techniques.
- A radiographer working in an out-patient setting is working with undergraduate learners from a local university on placement. During these five-week full-time blocks, the senior is responsible for facilitating their learning on a day-to-day basis.
- A speech and language therapist working in oncology is joined by an experienced practitioner undertaking a specialist practice-based module as part of an MSc programme.
- A physiotherapist is involved in developing and delivering an induction programme for therapy assistants in collaboration with occupational-therapy colleagues.

In these scenarios, practitioners are involved in:

- teaching/instructing learners how to perform specific tasks;
- organising learning opportunities and facilitating the learning process;
- assessing to what extent learning has occurred;
- giving feedback on newly acquired skills and abilities to help learners improve further.

This list is not exhaustive but it illustrates the integral and vital role of health practitioners in practice-based education and learning.

EXPLORATORY REFLECTION 2.4

- Think about the ways in which you are involved with educating others as part of your daily work. Look back to the quotation from Billet (1999) on p. 17. On reflection, what learning-related experiences (formal or informal) have you had that have played a part in preparing you for a role as a practice-based educator?

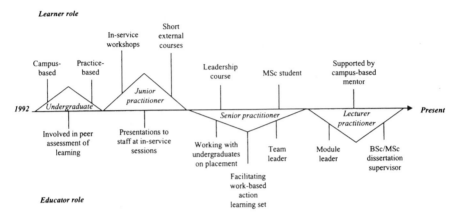

Figure 2.3. Time line of learning-related experiences.

- Construct a time line to help you think about this. Above the line mark all the times you have been in the role of learner, and below the line all the times you have taken on the role of educator in some way. We have provided a simple example in Figure 2.3 above, but make your own time line as detailed as possible.

Current issues influencing practice-based education

Over the last few years, there has been an increasing emphasis on the importance of practice-education placements and the need to assure their quality. The Department of Health and other bodies have published a succession of key documents. Some of these are listed in Table 2.1, and short summaries are provided below. Depending on your context, they highlight the relevance of each document to your work as a practice-based educator. In the reference list at the end of the chapter are the relevant Web addresses to enable you to explore the history and context of the summary points in more detail if you wish. The Department of Health's website (http://www.DH.gov.uk) is an important starting point to get information on the most recent developments relating to the quality review of health-professional courses.

Quality review of health-professional courses

University courses are subject to a wide range of quality reviews. This is particularly true for health-professional courses. The Quality Assurance Agency (QAA) has been reviewing the quality of courses in HEIs for the last decade. The NHS contracted with the QAA to carry out a new round of major review

Table 2.1. Key developments and documents associated with practice-based education

2005	HPC confirms standards for CPD
	College of Occupational Therapy adopts CSP ACE model and launches Accreditation of Practice Placement Educators (APPLE)
2004	HPC *Consultation on CPD*
	Launch of Accreditation of Practice-Based Educators (ACE) scheme by Chartered Society of Physiotherapy
	HPC *Standards of Education*
2003	QAA major reviews of health-professional courses
2002	QAA code of practice for placement learning
2001	*Placements in Focus/Preparation of Teachers and Mentors* Workforce Development Confederations established *Working Together – Learning Together*
2000	*NHS Plan* *A Health Service of all the Talents* *Meeting the Challenge*

of all health-professional courses between 2003 and 2006. The major change from previous QAA reviews is that 'placement learning' will be subject to equal scrutiny alongside university-based learning.

There are variations in the quality process in different parts of the UK. The QAA's website sets out details of enhancement-led institutional review (ELIR), which is one of five main elements of a new approach to quality in Scotland. It also gives details of institutional review in Wales and institutional audit in Northern Ireland. The documents and strategies described below illustrate the fundamental principles underlying the different approaches.

In addition to QAA review, health-professional courses are monitored by their own institutional quality-review procedures, by the professional and statutory bodies and by their strategic health authorities. Despite the heavy emphasis on the quality of academic provision, never before have practice placements been subject to the same scrutiny. Previous lack of quality review of practice-based learning is difficult to justify, since it forms a substantial and integral part of most health-professional courses, often contributing to the academic outcome (degree award). Little attention has been focused on the practice environment or the educational skills of clinical practitioners responsible for facilitating and assessing students. One reason for this is that placements in most health professions are in short supply and there has been concern that this position should not be exacerbated.

Major review of health-professional courses occurs once every five years. Ongoing quality monitoring and enhancement (OQME) occur in the interim between one review and the next. In England, these and any initial approval of courses are part of the Partnership Quality Assurance Framework for Healthcare Education, http://www.qaa.ac.uk/health/framework/default.asp. This involves collaborative working between the Department of Health with education commissioners, education providers (HEIs and placement providers), Nursing and Midwifery Council (NMC), Health Professions Council (HPC) and service users. Through this process, education commissioners and regulators satisfy themselves that the quality of education programmes provided by HEIs and placement providers is maintained and improved.

Code of practice (QAA, 2001a)

This QAA (2001a) code of practice forms part the review of health-professional courses placement learning and seals the place of placements in future quality-review policies and processes. In practical terms, the code itemises the expectations of practice learning and responsibilities of the stakeholders.

EXPLORATORY REFLECTION 2.5

Read the latest version of the code of the QAA practice for placement learning.

- How far do you think the section relating to placement providers is being fulfilled? Are practice-based educators in your service being adequately supported and prepared?
- What changes (if any) could you suggest in your service?

A Health Service of all the Talents (DH, 2000a)

- consultation document based on a review of workforce planning;
- includes 'recognition of the need to build on and develop partnership with those providing training and education for the NHS workforce and with relevant regulatory bodies';
- emphasises the need for genuine multiprofessional education and new types of healthcare workers;
- highlights the need for team working and flexible approaches to working;
- places a 'clear responsibility on individual employers and Workforce Development Confederations to establish good quality clinical placements'.

NHS Plan (DH, 2000b)

- intended to give the people of Britain a health service fit for the twenty-first century, a health service designed around the patient;

- key amongst its proposals is an intention to increase numbers of nurses and therapists;
- also proposes better use be made of investment in CPD of staff with greater emphasis being placed on accredited workplace learning.

Meeting the Challenge (DH, 2000c)

- sets out a plan to put allied health professions at the forefront of the NHS;
- highlights action on increased recruitment and improved retention of staff including plans to fund return to work for qualified staff after a career break;
- encourages employers to work with consortia (for example Workforce Development Confederations) and education providers (for example HEIs) to ensure adequate numbers of high-quality practice placements for students;
- identifies education as a key part of every professional practitioner's role – ensuring the next generation of professionals is competent to practice;
- urges better recognition of the practice-based educator's role through more systematic organisation, staffing and management practices.

EXPLORATORY REFLECTION 2.6

Read Section 4 of DH (2000c).

Select one of the bullet points listed in the summary above and find out what progress has been made towards achieving this goal since publication in 2000.

Working Together – Learning Together (DH, 2001)

- sets out a 'vision' for lifelong learning in the NHS;
- embraces core values such as effective communication, team working and understanding of the NHS;
- emphasises early interprofessional working and 'common learning';
- emphasises the need for practice placements to be of consistent quality with structured placement supervision and support;
- joint appointments between HEIs and the health sector are recommended;
- promotes links between placement standards and clinical-governance arrangements;
- promotes widening access to professional education for disadvantaged groups and more flexible career pathways enabling students or qualified staff to move more easily between programmes.

Placements in Focus (ENB & DH, 2001a)

- provides practical guidance to enhance the quality and innovative development of practice placements;
- expands and makes more explicit existing guidance and standards for students' placements.

A complementary document published at the same time (*Preparation of Mentors and Teachers*: ENB & DH, 2001b) contains specific guidance to aid the implementation and improve support to students on placement. The two documents stress shared responsibility for ensuring quantity and quality of practice-placement provision to support and educate the next generation of healthcare professionals. The document also notes that students have a responsibility to be active participants in their own learning and make the best use of learning opportunities in their practice areas. The importance of practice-based educators having appropriate experience but also appropriate preparation for their role in relation to educational programmes is stressed. This is linked to the need for time being made available for practitioners to fulfil the role.

Although nursing-focused, both documents contain many sound ideas in relation to placement learning and provision that are transferable to learning within the allied health professions.

EXPLORATORY REFLECTION 2.7

Scan ENB & DH (2001a).

- Identify one idea that could be/has been adopted in your setting to improve placement provision.
- Explain the potential/actual benefits.

In many of these articles and documents, there is reference to interprofessional working, multiprofessional working, shared learning and common core. The variation in terminology may lead to misunderstanding and confusion and may account for some slowness in interprofessional initiatives being put into action. There is a broad spectrum of aims in relation to implementation. At one end of the spectrum are staunch supporters of individual professional identities and expertise who recognise the need for effective teamwork and communication. At the other end are those with a vision of the generic therapist. In any discussion around the merits of interprofessional working, it is important that participants understand each other's working definitions to avoid being at cross purposes (Barr, 2002).

The role of Workforce Development Directorates

- bring together NHS and non-NHS employers (for example local authorities, private and voluntary) to plan and develop the whole healthcare workforce;

- have a key role in increasing staff numbers, changing training and education patterns and tackling recruitment and retention issues;
- commission and manage quality-assured education and training;
- have responsibility for practice placements and work with HEIs to ensure sufficient numbers of suitable placements are available and modernisation aims are achieved;
- in partnership with HEIs and professional bodies they ensure all practice-based learning environments meet specific government targets, are quality-assured and responsive to student evaluation and feedback;
- promote interprofessional learning.

Framework for Higher Education Qualifications (QAA, 2001b)

This framework aims to increase public confidence in academic standards. It is designed to ensure consistent use of qualification titles. Its stated aims are to:

- enable employers, schools, parents, prospective students and others to understand the achievements and attributes represented by the main qualification titles;
- maintain international comparability of standards, especially in the European context, to ensure international competitiveness and to facilitate student and graduate mobility;
- assist learners to identify potential progression routes, particularly in the context of lifelong learning;
- assist HEIs, their external examiners and the Agency's reviewers by providing important points of reference for setting and assessing standards.

Benchmark standards (QAA, 2001c)

These are intended to describe the nature and characteristics of programmes of study and training in health care. Wording in the document contributes to the formation of learning outcomes for academic and practice components of courses along with the HPC (2003) standards of proficiency, which all practitioners must meet in order to become registered, and continue to meet in order to maintain their registration.

Special Educational Needs and Disabilities Act (SENDA) (DH, 1995)

This Act forms Part 4 of the Disability Discrimination Act (DH, 1995). It has important implications for educators in HEIs and practice-based placements. All students are covered by the Act, and all institutions must ensure students with disabilities have equal opportunities while on practice placements. SENDA legislation aims to ensure students with disabilities have equal opportunity both to benefit from and contribute to campus-based and practice-based learning. Guidelines produced by the Chartered Society of Physiotherapy (2004a, 2004b) contain some useful suggestions for supporting learners in the practice setting, and many of the learning and teaching strategies suggested are examples of good practice in any professional context.

Accreditation of practice-based educators

In 2004, the Chartered Society of Physiotherapy began to offer members recognition for their valuable role as practice-based educators through the Accreditation of Clinical Educators (ACE) scheme (CSP, 2004b). At the official launch of the scheme, the then advisor to the DH Learning and Personal Development Division commented:

> I envisage ACE becoming one of the most important tools in enabling [therapists] to continue lifelong learning and contribute to the knowledge and skills agenda. (Wilson, 2004)

A system of accreditation will:

- contribute to continuing professional development of individual practitioners in relation to their role as practice-based educators;
- provide a baseline standard in this crucial aspect of healthcare practice;
- be influential in raising clinical standards.

Eligibility for accreditation is based on evidence of achievement of a set of common learning outcomes. HEIs facilitate practitioners to work towards accreditation, either through formal courses or recognition of experiential learning. The Chartered Society of Physiotherapy approves both routes. Successful participants are eligible for accredited status. A national system of accreditation avoids the possibility of individual clinical educators having to be accredited by several HEIs when they take students from more than one institution. ACE is fully congruent with the current emphasis on interprofessional initiatives, in that courses or programmes linked to accredited status are open to clinicians from a variety of health disciplines. The College of Occupational Therapists (COT, 2005) has adapted ACE in the form of 'Accreditation of Practice Placement Educators' (APPLE), and other professions have expressed interest.

Currently, accreditation is voluntary rather than mandatory. Full details of the ACE and APPLE frameworks are available on the CSP and COT websites and, although copyrighted, can readily be adopted by other health professions in the UK and elsewhere.

EXPLORATORY REFLECTION 2.8

- Have any of your colleagues applied for and achieved accreditation as a practice-based educator?
- If so, discuss the process with them; what do they consider has been the impact on their practice as an educator?
- Consider the pros and cons of applying for accreditation as a practice-based educator yourself.
- If possible, look at the relevant documentation and think about how this book might assist your application.

Summary

This chapter has introduced definitions, models and context of practice-based learning. Important points to consider are:

- There are differences between, and within, professions in terminology and models of practice-based learning.
- The profile and importance of practice-based learning and practice-based educators is higher now than ever before and continues to develop in response to various political and professional drivers.
- Developing the necessary knowledge and skills for good practice as an educator is a learning process in itself, requiring appropriate facilitation and support.

Now complete the portfolio sheet for Chapter 2.

- Check how often you are involved in activities associated with achieving quality in practice-based education.
- Consider whether now is the time for you to pursue recognition as a practice-based educator through accreditation.
- Identify your continued-development needs.
- Reassess your confidence in relation to Chapter 2's learning outcomes, including any personal learning outcomes you identified for yourself.
- Complete your action plan.

Finally, discuss the different ways in which Chapter 2 has helped you to think about your role as a practice-based educator. What reflective purposes has the chapter served for you?

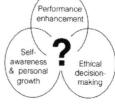

Portfolio Sheet – Practice-based learning and healthcare quality

Activities associated with achieving quality in practice-based education	Frequency of involvement			Existing evidence to suggest you should pursue the opportunity to gain recognition as a practice-based educator through accreditation	Development need?	
	Regularly	Occasionally	Never		YES	NO
Being involved in a variety of learning relationships in your practice environment.	☐	☐	☐		☐	☐
Looking for opportunities to broaden the scope of your practice-based education activity (different types and levels).	☐	☐	☐		☐	☐
Recording your own history and achievements as a learner and educator.	☐	☐	☐		☐	☐
Regularly accessing Web-based resources to keep abreast of policy related to healthcare and education.	☐	☐	☐		☐	☐
Acting as a change agent in the evolution of practice-based education in your practice environment.	☐	☐	☐		☐	☐

Sufficient evidence? YES ☐ NO ☐

Chapter 2's Learning Outcomes

	I am confident I can do this	I am not sure I can do this
1. Discuss the range of learning that takes place in your own practice context.	☐	☐
2. Identify key stages in the evolution of practice-based education in your own profession.	☐	☐
3. Identify terminology and models related to practice-based learning used in your own and other health professions with whom you work and collaborate.	☐	☐
4. Explain the reasons for the growing importance of practice-based learning and practice-based educators in terms of healthcare quality.	☐	☐
5. Discuss existing factors that influence further development of practice-based learning and the practice-based educator's role.	☐	☐

Personal learning outcomes for Chapter 2

Confident   Not sure

☐   ☐

ACTION PLAN

Bibliography

**Barr H (2002) *Inter-professional Education Today, Yesterday and Tomorrow: A Review*. London: Learning and Teaching Support Network for Health Sciences and Practice.

**Billet S (1999) Guided learning in the workplace. In Boud D, Garrick J (eds), *Understanding Learning at Work*, London: Routledge.

*Chartered Society of Physiotherapy (2004a) *Guidance: Supporting Disabled Physiotherapy Students on Clinical Placement*. London: CSP.

Chartered Society of Physiotherapy (2004b) Accreditation of Practice-Based Educators (ACE) <http://www.csp.org.uk/membergroups/educators/ace.cfm> (accessed 27 February 2006).

College of Occupational Therapists (2005) Accreditation of Practice Placement Educators (APPLE) <http://www.cot.org.uk/public/introduction/intro.php> (accessed 27 February 2006).

*Cross V (1994) From clinical supervisor to clinical educator: too much to ask? *Physiotherapy*, 80(9), 609–611.

Department of Health (1995) Disability Discrimination Act 1995 (c. 50), <http://www.opsi.gov.uk/acts/acts1995/1995050.htm> (accessed 27 February 2006).

Department of Health (2000a) A Health Service of all Talents: Developing the NHS Workforce, <http://www.doh.gov.uk/wfprconsult/> (accessed 27 February 2006).

Department of Health (2000b) NHS Plan 2000. A Plan for Investment. A Plan for Reform, <http://www.dh.gov.uk> (accessed 27 February 2006).

Department of Health (2000c) Meeting the Challenge: A Strategy for the Allied Health Professions, <http://www.doh.gov.uk/meetingthechallenge/> (accessed 27 February 2006).

Department of Health (2001) Working Together – Learning Together. A Framework for Life long Learning in the NHS, <http://www.doh.gov.uk/pdfs/teachers.pdf> (accessed 27 February 2006).

English National Board for Nursing, Midwifery and Health Visiting and Department of Health (2001a) Placements in Focus: Guidelines for Education in Practice for Health Professions, <http://www.doh.gov.uk/pdfs/places.pdf> (accessed 27 February 2006).

English National Board for Nursing, Midwifery and Health Visiting and Department of Health (2001b) *Preparation of Mentors and Teachers*. London: ENB & DH.

HPC (2003) Standards of Proficiency, <http://www.hpcuk.org/education/index.htm> (accessed 27 February 2006).

HPC (2004a) Consultation on CPD, <http://www.hpc-uk.org/consultation/cpd.htm> (accessed 27 February 2006).

HPC (2004b) Standards of Education, <http://www.hpc-uk.org/> (accessed 27 February 2006).

Lewin K (1951) *Field Theory in Social Science*. New York: Harper and Row.

Quality Assurance Agency for Higher Education (2001a) QAA Code of Practice for Placement Learning, <http://www.qaa.ac.uk/academicinfrastructure/codeOfPractice/section9/default.asp> (accessed 27 February 2006).

Quality Assurance Agency for Higher Education (2001b) Framework for Higher Education Qualifications, <http://www.qaa.ac.uk/academicinfrastructure/FHEQ/default.asp> (accessed 27 February 2006).

Quality Assurance Agency for Higher Education (2001c) Subject benchmarks for health professions, <http://www.qaa.ac.uk/academicinfrastructure/benchmark/health/default.asp> (accessed 27 February 2006).

Wilson F (2004) CSP raises clinical standards with ACE scheme. Press release, 5 March 2004. <http://www.csp.org.uk/search/result.cfm?itemID=51499f72EB031 F9059DE3A1957B0D1F1&module=news&cat=837AC15007128018EB6C4134A FE1>.

Further reading

Department for Education and Skills (2002) Providing Work Placements for Disabled Students: A Good Practice Guide for Further and Higher Education Institutions (Ref: DfES/0024/2002), Nottingham, <http://www.shef.ac.uk/~md1djw/HCP-disability/dyslexia/workplacment.html> (accessed 27 February 2006).

Martin H (2005) Do placement visits offer value for money? *British Journal of Occupational Therapy*, 68(4), 186–187.

** Suitable for readers who wish to examine concepts at a more detailed or advanced level.
* Suitable for readers looking for something to stimulate ideas in a straightforward way.

3 MULTIPLE ROLES OF THE PRACTICE-BASED EDUCATOR

Introduction   Despite increased recognition of its importance, the role of the practice-based educator in its broadest sense is often underestimated in terms of its variety and complexity. This chapter explores the role in detail and identifies desirable qualities for practice-based educators.

PREPARATORY REFLECTION   Working through this chapter should enable you to achieve the learning outcomes listed below. Before continuing, consider how confident you feel now in relation to these outcomes and tick the appropriate box beside each one. Are there any personal learning outcomes you would like to add to the list?

Learning outcomes

	I am confident I can do this	I am not sure I can do this
1. Discuss the personal qualities that you think are needed for the successful fulfilment of your role as a practice-based educator both now and in the future.	☐	☐
2. Analyse your activities as an educator in relation to the following three key elements of the practice-based educator's role:		

	I am confident I can do this	I am not sure I can do this

- o facilitator of learning;   ☐   ☐
- o assessor of learning and performance;   ☐   ☐
- o evaluator of the learning experience.   ☐   ☐

3. Identify those aspects of the role in which you feel:
   - o most comfortable;   ☐   ☐
   - o least comfortable;   ☐   ☐
   - o you have a definite development need   ☐   ☐

   and explain the reasons underlying your choice.

Think about any personal outcomes that you would like to add to this list and make a note of them.

What is the role of the practice-based educator?

In Chapter 2, we examined the wider context of practice-based education. Three main functions emerged:

1. supporting and helping people to learn in practice-based settings;
2. maintaining standards of clinical performance and enhancing the quality of healthcare delivery;
3. enriching the overall practice-based learning experience.

Here we consider the ways in which practice-based educators fulfil these three functions, and subsequent chapters will expand on the ideas introduced here.

EXPLORATORY REFLECTION 3.1

So, what is the role of the practice-based educator? Enlist the help of a small group of colleagues from different health professions if possible, and exchange ideas. Try to think as laterally and creatively as possible.

- Record the responses on a flip chart or large sheet of paper. Accept every response at this preliminary stage and do not discuss the various ideas and proposals.
- When no more ideas are forthcoming, discuss each response and then organise them into categories.
- Compare the results of your discussion with the ideas in the rest of the chapter.

Essentially, the role of the practice-based educator is that of communicator. However, your thoughts and discussions should have confirmed the com-

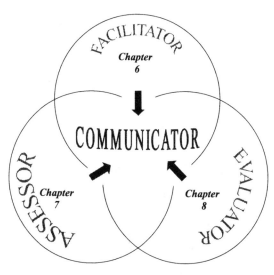

Figure 3.1. Role dimensions of the practice-based educator.

plexity and multidimensional nature of this communication role. Here we describe three key dimensions (Figure 3.1); they are facilitation, assessment and evaluation. Subsequent chapters elaborate on each role dimension as shown in Figure 3.1.

> The move to a more student-centred view of learning has required a fundamental shift in the role of the teacher. No longer is the teacher seen predominantly as a dispenser of information or walking tape recorder but rather as a facilitator or manager of the students' learning . . . The more responsibility given to the student the greater the shift in the teacher role. (Harden & Crosby, 2000, p. 339)

The practice-based educator as a facilitator of learning

In Exploratory Reflection 3.1 you may have identified a large number of roles that can be grouped within the dimension of facilitation. Figure 3.2 illustrates four key elements within facilitation: professional, resource guide, mentor and manager. We will look more closely at each of these in turn.

The facilitator as a professional

Working as a health professional is integral to the role of the practice-based educator. This includes your activities as a healthcare practitioner and also a teacher. As a practitioner, you present as an expert to students, patients and other healthcare professionals. As such, you may be a role model to any of

- Motivator
- Enabler
- Lecturer
- Tutor
- Demonstrator
- Negotiator

- Expert
- Role model
- Performance coach
- Advocate

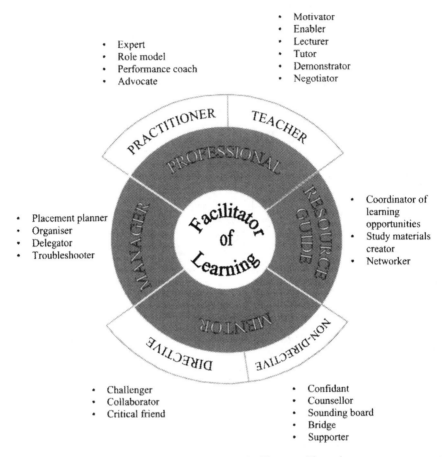

- Placement planner
- Organiser
- Delegator
- Troubleshooter

- Coordinator of learning opportunities
- Study materials creator
- Networker

- Challenger
- Collaborator
- Critical friend

- Confidant
- Counsellor
- Sounding board
- Bridge
- Supporter

Figure 3.2. The practice-based educator as a facilitator of learning.

these learners. As you actively re-evaluate their own professional practice, you help learners understand the value of reflective practice, and justify your status as a role model.

Practitioners also act as coaches, setting objectives to help improve existing performance as opposed to acquiring new knowledge or skills (Klasen & Clutterbuck, 2002). Lastly, as a practitioner, you may act as an advocate and intermediary between students and HEI tutors, as you do for patients in dealing with other health professionals and organisations. You may also advocate for other practitioners for whom you may have educational responsibility.

As a teacher, you are first and foremost a motivator and enabler. Biggs (1999, p. 61) describes the motivator function as communicating to students the need to learn, and suggests that 'motivation is the product of good teaching, not its prerequisite'.

However, learners also need to know that achievement is within their reach and that their efforts to learn will be supported. Other aspects include acting as a tutor or lecturer to large or small groups of individuals, such as students, other health professionals or patient-support groups. The practice-based educator is also a demonstrator of new skills to junior staff and student health professionals.

The facilitator as a resource guide

In this aspect of the role you may:

- *coordinate* a series of learning opportunities such as demonstrations and visits by student health professionals to other departments and service locations;
- *develop study material* to help learners, for example hand outs, producing overhead projection transparencies or multimedia presentations for larger groups using software packages such as PowerPoint;
- guide learners and others to resources and networks that can support their experience. For students and junior health professionals this could mean directing them to appropriate journals for key articles. For patients and carers it could be highlighting the availability of information sheets, booklets or support material available from organisations such as the Parkinson's Disease Society, British Diabetic Association, The Arthritis Council etc.

The facilitator as a mentor

Enabling people to be productive learners without fear of failure and at the same time challenging their assumptions, previous behaviours and existing knowledge are important aspects of the mentor's role. This may involve collaborating as a fellow learner or acting as a critical friend to prompt critical reflection from learners on their own performance. In a less directive capacity, you may be regarded by the learner as a confidant or counsellor, although always mindful of the need to know when to seek further help from a professional counsellor if it appears indicated. You may provide a sounding board for evolving ideas or a bridge to new understanding. At any stage, the practice-based educator may offer learning, social and personal support to learners at different times in the learning experience. The practice-based educator may also provide peer support, particularly if involved in practice-based education activities involving colleagues.

The role of mentor can be a difficult one to get right and can sometimes feel like a heavy responsibility. Educators and learners work closely together, and sometimes friendships develop. It is important always to be able to step back from this relationship to provide enough distance to avoid compromising other dimensions of your role, such as those of assessor and evaluator.

It is important to get the balance absolutely right between this aspect of the facilitator's role and the role of assessor and evaluator.

The facilitator as a manager

There is no doubt that things go best when they are managed well, and practice-based learning is no exception. This aspect of the facilitator role involves planning learning experiences, such as student placements, or planning a learning experience for a patient and a carer. It may involve organising a series of in-service lectures or a series of learning events. This aspect of the role includes management of all organisational and administrative components of the learning experience, and at the same time being cognisant of and responsive to any change in circumstances in the workplace, such as staff sickness, fluctuating patient caseloads and other service demands that may directly or indirectly impact on the learning experience. Within this role, you may engage in collaboration with other educators in the practice setting or liaise with members of higher-education institutions. Planning a learning experience in detail may involve collaboration with a large number of people who will contribute to the learning experience from both inside and outside the workplace. Finally, you must be a troubleshooter, solving small and potentially larger problems that may occur during the course of a learning experience. These need to be anticipated and minimised in order to avoid undermining the quality of the learning experience.

The practice-based educator as an assessor

Assessment involves making judgements about learners' abilities, performance and competence at different times and for a variety of reasons. This role is examined in detail in Chapter 7.

EXPLORATORY REFLECTION 3.2

Think about the sort of assessment judgements you make as an educator.

- What do you make judgements about?
- Why is it necessary to assess? You might find it useful to think about this in terms of benefits to the learner, the employer, the profession and the university or college.
- When do you make assessment judgements?
- How do you make assessment judgements?

When you have completed this activity, see where your analysis fits with the assessor role summarised in Figure 3.3.

It will be clear from Figure 3.3 that assessment judgements fall into two main categories based on why the assessment is being carried out, that is its

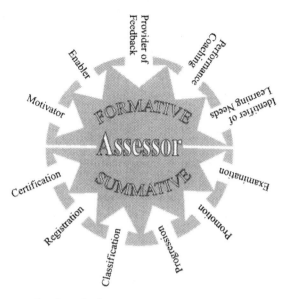

Figure 3.3. The practice-based educator as an assessor.

purpose. In relation to the first category (formative), preparing for assessment judgements is a key function, for example by providing feedback or coaching. In relation to the second category (summative), activity centres on the actual judgement process, as we explain below.

Formative purposes: When assessment takes place during a course of study, or a learning event such as a treatment session, and learners are able to benefit from feedback on their performance, then the purpose is formative. For the learner, formative assessment should motivate and encourage, both in anticipation of the event and by the feedback that is given subsequently in which strengths and weaknesses can be identified and discussed constructively. In addition, it should give some guidelines on how performance might be improved. It is clear from this that there is a good deal of overlap between activities associated with learning facilitation and those associated with formative assessment.

EXPLORATORY REFLECTION 3.3

Think back over your recent activities with students, patients/clients, colleagues, carers etc.

Can you identify occasions when your purpose was to:

- motivate someone to do their best?
- improve specific elements in performance of a skill?

- identify some specific learning needs to be addressed in a learning programme or event?
- support someone through a difficult learning situation?

Now ask yourself:

- Who does these things for me?
- Do I do them for myself?

Summative purposes: When it is necessary to label or rank learners, or provide an official indicator of achievement, then the purpose is summative. This aspect of the assessor's role will involve you in gathering evidence of achievement to meet the needs of a variety of stakeholders in professional education at all levels. Your judgements may influence, for example, undergraduates' eligibility for state registration and/or degree classification or their progression from one year of their course to the next. Your judgement might also influence a junior colleague's promotion to a more senior grade. For learners undertaking post-registration courses, your judgement may influence their certification. As part of your role, you may also be involved in the examination of undergraduate or postgraduate students in the practice setting.

For employers, professional bodies and the general public, there must be confidence that standards are being maintained so the public can be assured of optimum levels of competence to practise. For HEIs, summative assessment serves to monitor individual students' performance as well as the overall success of a programme of study.

The two main purposes of assessment are not necessarily mutually exclusive and some methods of assessment might fulfil both purposes simultaneously. Chapter 7 explores the elements of your assessor role in detail and describes a variety of methods you might use.

The practice-based educator as an evaluator

The third dimension of the practice-based educator's role is that of evaluator, and the elements of this dimension are shown in Figure 3.4. An important question to ask at this point is, 'What is the difference between assessment and evaluation?' Educators in the United Kingdom use the terms 'assessment' and 'evaluation' to describe different functions (Freeman & Lewis, 1998).

Assessment focuses on people's learning. We look for evidence of learning in their behaviour (oral, written or practical). This enables us to make judgements about what they can or cannot do, and to make inferences about what they might be able to do in the future.

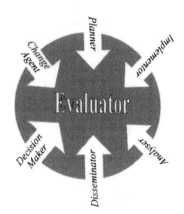

Figure 3.4. The practice-based educator as an evaluator.

> **Evaluation** focuses on how the various aspects of the learning experience perform – in other words, the performance of the provider and the provision. This enables us to develop strategies for improving the quality of, for example, placement planning, content and delivery.

Unless all aspects of the learning experience are evaluated, there is little hope of improving its quality. Evaluation may involve learners, educators, peers and, in the case of undergraduate and postgraduate students, colleagues from HEIs. It involves several activities, as shown in Figure 3.4. Evaluation must be planned in terms of:

- what aspects of the learning experience will be evaluated;
- how it will be done;
- who will carry it out;
- when it will occur.

Then evaluation must be carried out, results analysed, findings disseminated and discussed with relevant and interested individuals. If findings indicate that the learning experience should be changed or modified to improve its quality or impact, then as a final stage in the evaluation process, relevant changes must be agreed and implemented. The evaluation of learning experiences is considered in depth in Chapter 8.

Rewards for the practice-based educator

We should not leave our exploration of the practice-based educator without considering some of the rewards that this role can bring. The perspectives of educators in health care have identified a number of personal rewards (Paterson, 1994; Gwyer, 1993), for example:

To teach learners I must keep my knowledge and skills up to date.

Interaction with the learner causes me to constantly analyse the care I'm giving my patients.

The learners stimulate me to learn more.

[I enjoy] making a difference, watching them grow, learning from them and with them.

Providing high-quality learning experiences based on sound evaluation can benefit the workplace, for example by increased recruitment and heightened national profile as a clinical education centre. In addition, the professional profiles of practitioners themselves may be enhanced through accreditation as educators. You may have decided to use the activities in this book as a means of helping you achieve this. Perhaps most importantly, by valuing, encouraging and nurturing the learning capabilities of other health professionals, you are empowering them to bring about change and produce real improvements in the effectiveness of clinical practice and the quality of health service delivery.

The learner's perspective

As mentioned previously, the role of the practice-based educator is multidimensional and as such requires many different qualities. It is interesting to examine what importance learners attach to different elements of the educator's role. Cross (1995) compares, in terms of behaviours, perceptions of the ideal clinical educator held by learners, clinical educators and academic tutors. Interestingly, the academic tutors' perceptions were different from those of the learners and the clinical educators.

EXPLORATORY REFLECTION 3.4

Below is a list of 43 educator behaviours. The list is based on early, but still relevant, work by Emery (1984) involving health-professional students, who identified them as important and grouped them into broad categories. Rank the categories in terms of their relative importance for you. For example, if you feel that the category 'Teaching behaviours' contains the most important set of characteristics, put number 1 against that. If you feel that 'Professional-skills behaviours' is the next most important set, put 2 against that, and so on.

1. Communication behaviours   *Rank*

□

    a. Makes himself/herself understood

    b. Provides useful feedback

    c. Is an active listener

    d. Provides positive feedback on performance
    e. Communicates in a non-threatening manner
    f. Openly and honestly reveals perceptions held of the learner
    g. Provides timely feedback
    h. Is open in discussing issues with the learner
    i. Teaches in an interactive way; encourages dialogue
    j. Provides feedback in private

2. *Interpersonal-relations behaviours*   *Rank*

□

    a. Establishes an environment in which the learner feels
       comfortable
    b. Provides appropriate support for the learner's concerns,
       frustrations and anxieties
    c. Empathises with the learner
    d. Demonstrates a genuine concern for patients
    e. Introduces the learner to others as a professional
    f. Demonstrates a positive regard for the learner as a person

3. *Professional-skills behaviours*   *Rank*

□

    a. Employs physical therapy practice with competence
    b. Demonstrates professional behaviour as a member of the
       healthcare team
    c. Demonstrates systematic approach to problem solving
    d. Explains physiological basis of physical therapy treatment
    e. Explains physiological basis of physical therapy evaluation
    f. Demonstrates the appropriate role of physical therapy as
       part of total health care
    g. Serves as an appropriate role model
    h. Manages own time well
    i. Demonstrates leadership among peers

4. *Teaching behaviours*   *Rank*

□

    a. Allows the learner progressive, appropriate independence
    b. Is available to the learner
    c. Makes the formal evaluation a constructive process
    d. Makes an effective learning experience out of situations
       as they arise
    e. Plans effective learning experiences
    f. Provides a variety of patients

g. Questions/coaches in such a way as to help the learner
  to learn
h. Points out discrepancies in the learner's performance
i. Provides unique learning experiences
j. Demonstrates the relationship between academic knowledge
  and clinical practice
k. Is accurate in documenting learner evaluation
l. Helps the learner to define specific objectives for the
  clinical-education experience
m. Observes performance in a discreet manner
n. Schedules regular meetings with the learner
o. Plans learning experiences before the learner arrives
p. Manages the learner's time well
q. Is timely in documenting the learner's evaluation
r. Is perceived as a consistent extension of the academic
  programme

Ask a colleague and a learner to rank categories 1–4. Do you agree with each other? How do you account for any differences that exist between you?

Categories	Self	Colleague	Learner
1. Communication	☐	☐	☐
2. Interpersonal relations	☐	☐	☐
3. Professional skills	☐	☐	☐
4. Teaching	☐	☐	☐

Now read Cross (1995) Perceptions of the ideal clinical educator in physiotherapy education. *Physiotherapy*, 81(9), 506–513. Compare the findings with your own views.

The impact of practice educators' behaviour on learners

Brookfield (1998) emphasises the importance of using our learners' eyes as a 'critically reflective lens'.

> Seeing our practice through learners' eyes helps us teach more responsively. Having a sense of what is happening to people as they grapple with the difficult, threatening, and exhilarating process of learning constitutes educators' primary information. Without this information it is hard to teach well. (Brookfield, 1998, p. 199)

The following comments were made by undergraduate health professionals following practice placements. They illustrate how influential a practice-based educator's behaviour can be on the learning process.

When discussing patient management, I was praised and encouraged if my understanding was good. If it wasn't good, I was encouraged to read books, notes, ask questions, etc. I was never harshly criticised but guided and corrected.

It was made perfectly clear that they were surprised by my lack of knowledge. I was constantly compared with learners who had previously been there on placement. I was told that my attitude was 'student-like' and unprofessional. This made me nervous, as I was unsure what I was doing wrong and unable to discuss it as I was too upset. It also made me paranoid as I didn't know who had said this about me and what I had done to deserve it.

Whilst being encouraged to ask questions, I found it difficult to approach my practice educator . . . and didn't want to push my luck by asking her to clarify points she had made.

My educator was up to date on the latest techniques and theories, so this gave me the opportunity to learn new skills as well as practise those learned in school.

EXPLORATORY REFLECTION 3.5

- Bearing in mind that each comment provides only one side of the story, what do the extracts above suggest to you about the developmental needs of the educators involved?
- Which of the desirable behaviours listed in Exploratory Reflection 3.4 do they demonstrate and which do they not demonstrate?

The importance of self-awareness Another important source of insight into our practice as educators is what Brookfield (1998, p. 197) describes as our 'autobiography as a learner'. Our experiences as learners often have a much more powerful and long-lasting influence on our behaviour as educators than any methods or advice we read about in books or hear from colleagues.

We may think we are teaching according to a widely accepted curricular or pedagogic model only to find, on reflection, that the foundations of how we work have been laid in our autobiographies as learners. In the face of crises or ambiguities, we fall back instinctively on memories from our times as learners to guide how we respond. (Brookfield, 1998, p. 198)

EXPLORATORY REFLECTION 3.6

- Recall three examples of experiences from your own practice-based education, either pre- or post-registration, that you feel had a positive effect on any aspect of your learning.
- Now consider experiences that you feel had a negative effect on your learning.

- Have any of these experiences contributed to or inhibited the development of your own skills as a practice-based educator? If you can, make a brief note below of some specific occasions when your past experience influenced your response to a learner.
- After completing the book, revisit these experiences and consider whether you would act any differently in light of your new knowledge.

Summary

This chapter has reviewed the importance and complexity of the practice-based educator's role. Important points to consider are:

- the practice-based educator's overarching role as a communicator comprises the dimensions of 'facilitator of learning', 'assessor' and 'evaluator';
- at times elements of these role dimensions may conflict with each other, for example that of mentor and assessor;
- in addition to its impact on learning and the quality of healthcare delivery, the role of practice-based educator brings personal rewards, for example personal fulfilment and empowerment and the possibility of professional accreditation;
- learners have clear expectations of practice-based educators;
- our behaviour as practice-based educators is influenced by our own personal experiences as learners.

Now complete the portfolio sheet for Chapter 3.

- Check how often you are involved in activities associated with the different role dimensions of the practice-based educator.
- Consider what evidence you have of your ability to fulfil ACCREDITATION OUTCOME I. Is it sufficient? If not, identify where the gaps lie and how they might be filled.
- Identify your continued development needs.
- Reassess your confidence in relation to Chapter 3's learning outcomes, including any personal learning outcomes that you set for yourself.
- Complete your action plan.

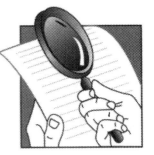

Finally, discuss the different ways in which Chapter 3 has helped you to think about your role as a practice-based educator. What reflective purposes has the chapter served for you?

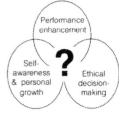

Portfolio Sheet – Multiple roles of the practice-based educator

Role dimensions and activities	Frequency of involvement			Existing evidence for ACCREDITATION OUTCOME I (give details)	Development need?	
	Regularly	Occasionally	Never		YES	NO

Facilitator of learning

Practitioner
Teacher
Resource guide
Non-directive mentor
Directive mentor
Manager

Assessor

Formative
Summative

Evaluator

Planner
Implementor
Analyser
Disseminator
Decision maker
Change agent

Describe the role and identify the attributes of the effective clinical educator

Sufficient evidence?   YES ☐   NO ☐

Chapter 3's Learning Outcomes

	I am confident I can do this	I am not sure I can do this
1. Discuss the personal qualities that you think are needed for the successful fulfilment of your role as a practice-based educator both now and in the future.	☐	☐
2. Analyse your activities in relation to the following three key elements of the practice-based educator's role:		
○ facilitator of learning	☐	☐
○ assessor of learning and performance	☐	☐
○ evaluator of the learning experience.	☐	☐
3. Identify those aspects of the role in which you feel:		
○ most comfortable	☐	☐
○ least comfortable	☐	☐
○ you have a definite development need and explain the reasons underlying your choice.	☐	☐

Personal learning outcomes for Chapter 3

Confident	Not sure
☐	☐

ACTION PLAN

Bibliography

Biggs J (1999) What the student does: teaching for enhanced learning. *Higher Education Research and Development*, 18(1), 57–75.

*Brookfield S (1998) Critically reflective practice. *The Journal of Continuing Education in the Health Professions*, 18, 197–205.

†Cross V (1995) Perceptions of the ideal clinical educator in physiotherapy education. *Physiotherapy*, 81(9), 506–513.

Emery MJ (1984) Effectiveness of the clinical instructor: students' perspective. *Physical Therapy*, 64(7), 1079–1083.

Freeman R, Lewis R (1998) *Planning and Implementing Assessment*. London: Kogan Page.

Gwyer J (1993) Rewards of teaching physical therapy students: clinical instructor's perspective. *Journal of Physical Therapy Education*, 7(2), 63–66.

*Harden RM, Crosby J (2000) The good teacher is more than a lecturer: the twelve roles of the teacher. *Medical Teacher*, 22(4), 334–347.

Klasen N, Clutterbuck D (2002) *Implementing Mentoring Schemes. A Practical Guide to Successful Programmes*. London: Butterworth-Heinemann.

Paterson B (1994) The view from within: perspectives of clinical teaching. *International Journal of Nursing Studies*, 31(4), 349–360.

Further reading

**Beckett D, Gough J (2004) Perceptions of professional identity: a story from paediatrics. *Studies in Continuing Education*, 26(2), 195–208.

**Pratt DD, Arseneau R, Collins JB (2001) Reconsidering 'good teaching' across the continuum of medical education. *The Journal of Continuing Education in the Health Professions*, 21(2), 70–81.

** Suitable for readers who wish to examine concepts at a more detailed or advanced level.
* Suitable for readers looking for something to stimulate ideas in a straightforward way.
† Included in the chapter as suggested reading.

4 THE PRACTICE-BASED LEARNING ENVIRONMENT: SOCIAL CONTEXT AND RELATIONSHIPS

Introduction In Chapter 2, we considered the wider context of practice-based learning, and in particular the impact of external influences on the organisational relationship between HEIs and the practice-based learning environment. In this chapter, we consider the practice-based learning environment in terms of individual educators and learners, and the social context within which they interact. We explore what factors set the scene for effective and fulfilling learning relationships.

PREPARATORY REFLECTION Working through this chapter should enable you to achieve the learning outcomes listed below. Before continuing, consider how confident you feel now in relation to these outcomes and tick the appropriate box beside each one. Are there any personal learning outcomes you would like to add to the list?

Learning outcomes

	I am confident I can do this	I am not sure I can do this
1. Analyse a range of healthcare settings in terms of the advantages and disadvantages they offer to learners and practice-based educators.	☐	☐

	I am confident I can do this	I am not sure I can do this
2. Identify and account for specific conflicts of interest you face as an educator and practitioner and analyse their potential impact on your relationship with learners.	☐	☐
3. Evaluate your effectiveness in building trusting relationships with learners in the practice setting.	☐	☐
4. Demonstrate your understanding of the effect of individual differences and needs on learners' and educators' beliefs about the learning process.	☐	☐
5. Identify aspects of legislation relevant to diversity and equal opportunities in learning and education.	☐	☐

Think about any personal outcomes that you would like to add to this list and make a note of them.

EXPLORATORY REFLECTION 4.1

Health professionals have varying perceptions of the task of practice-based education. These perceptions are influenced by their own experiences as learners. Think about some learning experiences that had (1) a positive outcome and (2) a negative outcome for you as a learner.

- Can you identify the reasons why the experiences were positive or negative?
- What were your thoughts and feelings at the time?
- What aspects of the experiences have stayed with you?

Compare your experiences with some of your colleagues. Do any common themes emerge? The chances are that some of the themes you identified are reflected in the following comments.

In a sense I easily felt I could say 'I don't understand that' without feeling that I *should* have understood it. I could openly say 'I don't understand' and we'd sit around and discuss it, before actually going to see the patient. I think if you're uncomfortable then you're not going to fully evaluate the situation and give your honest feeling about a situation. (Third-year undergraduate)

I think it's very important to give learners a good environment that they feel comfortable in. That's essential for them to be able to learn, so they feel comfortable in being able to ask questions. That's the most important thing you can do. (Practice-based educator)

The learning environment

These comments highlight the importance of the learning environment, which has been described as an interactive network of forces that influence students' learning outcomes (Dunn & Hansford, 1997) and a catalyst that governs learners' enthusiasm, commitment and receptiveness to the learning process (Lickman *et al.*, 1993; Simms *et al.*, 1990). Clinical practice is a challenging environment in which to learn and to facilitate learning. The enormity of its impact should not be underestimated. Figure 4.1 illustrates three sources of influence on learning environments.

Physical influences on the learning environment

The physical nature of environments can influence how people behave. In his influential work, the psychologist Maslow (1954) proposes a hierarchy of human needs that determine action. Needs at lower levels must be at least partially satisfied before those at higher levels can become significant motivators of action. Hence, the importance of meeting the basic security needs of learners before higher intellectual needs can be addressed; people feel more secure on familiar territory. Learners whose experiences straddle higher education and practice-based settings may be acutely aware of the different effects of each on their ability to engage with the learning process.

Educators based in HEIs can usually select from a variety of locations according to group size, course content and mode of delivery, for example lecture theatre, seminar room or clinical laboratory. Activities can be prepared in advance and learning resources easily accessed. The physical layout can be organised to influence interaction or convey different messages, for example the seating arrangements shown in Figure 4.2.

This degree of predictability is less likely in practice settings, which tend to be more dynamic and difficult to control. Developments in health- and social-care delivery have widened the range of learning environments, and this can pose difficulties for learners and educators (Hilton & Morris, 2001; Howe, 2001).

Figure 4.1. Influences on the learning environment.

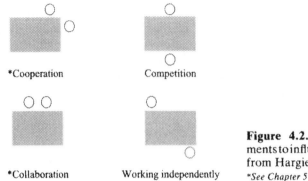

*Cooperation   Competition

*Collaboration   Working independently

Figure 4.2. Using seating arrangements to influence interaction (adapted from Hargie, 1991).
*See Chapter 5

I mean, this is the community; so you've got three people going to one patient ... Sometimes you've got a physiotherapist coming with you or a nurse. You may have a relative there as well; so that's up to six people in a room at a time. It does get a bit daunting having so many people there. (Second-year undergraduate)

EXPLORATORY REFLECTION 4.2

Figure 4.3 maps some of the healthcare settings in which practice-based learning takes place. From your own experience and that of colleagues, add to the range of settings shown.

- What do you consider to be the most controllable and uncontrollable elements in each case?
- What strategies have you used to help overcome any difficulties?

Psychosocial influences on the learning environment

Psychosocial influences can be defined as the influence of social factors on human interactive behaviour. Learning interactions have been described as 'psychosocial dramas' in which our best intentions often fall victim to 'unforeseen eventualities, serendipitous circumstances and individual idiosyncrasies' (Brookfield, 1986, p. 294). The nature of interactions between educators and learners is fundamental in determining the quality of learning experiences and maximising the potential of any learning environment.

The comments quoted at the start of the chapter both emphasise the need for learners to feel comfortable in the learning environment. As a social context, the practice setting demonstrates a variety of tensions and conflicts of interest or loyalty, likely to cause discomfort for educators and learners alike. For example, practice-based educators are torn between:

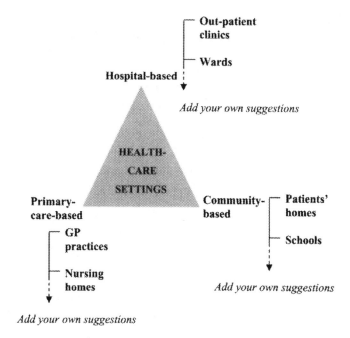

Figure 4.3. Healthcare settings for practice-based learning.

- providing a safe, effective service for healthcare users;
- creating challenging and stimulating opportunities for learners;
- devoting time to patients' clinical needs;
- allocating time to help learners develop their professional skills;
- acting as a learning facilitator;
- acting as an assessor of performance.

Learners may be torn between

- wanting to reveal their needs and uncertainties in order to receive help to develop;
- fear that by doing so they will appear incompetent and be labelled a failure;
- wanting to achieve the highest possible academic qualification;
- needing to be seen as competent for professional registration.

EXPLORATORY REFLECTION 4.3

- What specific conflicts of interest exist for you personally in your own practice setting?

- Do they differ from those experienced in other practice settings?
- What effect do they have on your relationship with learners?

The importance of trust in the learning environment

You may have come to the conclusion that one effect of environmental conflict is to undermine the trust between you and the learners with whom you interact. Trust is the foundation upon which the ultimate criterion of competence assessment – safety – rests (Ilott & Murphy, 1999). Learners at all levels (undergraduates, aspiring extended-scope practitioners and novice healthcare assistants) must demonstrate that they can be trusted to work safely with service users, even as they are learning. If not, they will require constant supervision. However, if learners must prove themselves trustworthy to educators, the converse also applies.

> Trust is crucial to facilitation . . . Real trust cannot be built where nothing is at stake and, without real trust, the depth of disclosure and reflection which leads to real, deep and personal learning will be restricted. (Hughes, 1999, pp. 36–37)

> Without a reasonably well-established sense of basic trust, it is difficult [for learners] to move ahead. (Daloz, 1999, p. 206)

Theories of facilitation emphasise the need for facilitators to work at building trusting relationships within the learning environment (Titchen, 2000; Heron, 1993; Brookfield, 1990). Most commentators agree that building a trusting relationship comes down to communication – dialogue between those directly involved. In Chapter 3, we identified a range of communication activities associated with learning facilitation. Look back to Figures 3.2 and 3.3 and you will see that certain activities stand out as particularly relevant to building trusting learning relationships, for example by acting as an advocate and intermediary for learners, offering support to validate learners' experience and perspectives, challenging learners' ideas and assumptions, encouraging them to reciprocate, helping learners reflect in safety by acting as a sounding board and by acting as a bridge towards new ways of thinking and acting.

EXPLORATORY REFLECTION 4.4

Make a list of learners with whom you and/or your colleagues interact on a regular basis. Your list might include:

- qualified practitioners undertaking work-based postgraduate modules;
- mature students on part-time undergraduate or qualifying master's programmes;
- traditional undergraduates on pre-registration placements;
- healthcare assistants working for vocational qualifications or foundation degrees;
- novice practitioners working through clinical rotations.

Discuss any obstacles that could exist to building trusting relationships in each case and some ways in which you might try to overcome them.

Cultural influences on the learning environment

> Culture is part and parcel of all that we do, all that we are, all that we can and might become ... in any one society there may be more than one culture or many small subcultures, the sum of which influences the individual. (Kidd, 2002, pp. 6, 11)

Culture has been described as one of the most complicated words in the English language (Williams, 1983). People themselves create culture, and what it stands for may be regarded as the central feature of all social life. It is described as a set of implicit and explicit guidelines or rules on how groups of people view the world and respond to it emotionally (Helman, 1994). It shows itself in behaviour and the way people communicate and interact (Coeling & Simms, 1993). Thus, culture helps to establish our sense of identity: how we think of ourselves as individuals, how we think of others and what we think they think of us. In particular, 'culture involves the majority of activities carried out in organisations' (Coeling & Simms, 1993, p. 47).

Subcultures

The term 'subculture' refers to a group that is in some way separate from the dominant culture. It has its own way of 'acting out' life, its own norms and values shared by a small proportion of a population. For example, the culture of speech and language therapy may be different from that of occupational therapy but, in addition, subspecialties within the same profession will have their own subculture.

> In reality, any given healthcare organisation can consist of as many subcultures as there are groups of people who work closely together and consider themselves 'our group'. (Coeling & Simms, 1993, p. 48)

Although some subcultures will conform, mostly, to the broader norms and values of the dominant group, 'deviant subcultures' actively reject them and may become alienated (Kidd, 2002). For example, major disagreement or resistance to imposed change can result in a deviant subgroup of individuals who 'play by their own rules' and attempt to subvert the dominant culture.

EXPLORATORY REFLECTION 4.5 Culture is a subtle force, rarely written down or communicated formally to newcomers. It is inferred from what group members say or do and is not obvious to the casual observer or participant (Coeling & Simms, 1993).

- What do you think are the implicit rules of the learning culture in your practice setting?
- Do you agree with the rules? Why? Why not?
- Does everyone follow the rules? What happens if they do not?
- How do you feel about yourself as a learner in your practice setting?
- What do you think about your colleagues as learners?
- What do you think is their opinion of you as a learner?
- What cultural messages do you think newcomers to your practice environment receive?
- To what extent does the learning culture in your practice setting embrace change and new ideas?

Cultural competence

Practitioners, service users and learners differ on such grouping factors as ethnicity, gender, sexual orientation, class, religion, disability and age. Increasing globalisation has enriched the mix of cultures and ethnic identities within learning communities in both higher education and healthcare practice. However:

> ... neither culture nor ethnicity are 'things' that people 'have'. They are, rather, complicated repertoires which people experience, use, learn and [act out] in their daily lives, upon which they draw for a sense of themselves and an understanding of their fellows. (Jenkins, 1999, p. 96)

The education of health professionals pays careful attention to the need for clinical practitioners to respect and respond to the range of values, beliefs and ways of 'being' of all service users and fellow workers. However, as the following anecdote from a colleague reveals, this is not always easy, even for experienced practitioners. As a white South African practitioner working with a black South African student, she received a valuable insight into her own practice.

> Here is a story about a humbling experience in lack of cultural competence I displayed. I thought I was quite good at treating people with respect – especially older adults. Then I went to see a patient with a black student. The student had been requested to interpret some questions about the elderly man's condition. I could not ask the questions myself because of a language barrier. The student proceeded to have a ten-minute conversation with the patient about how he was, where he came from and other aspects of his life before he went on to ask the clinical questions. My response was a sense of dismay at how rude I must have appeared on many occasions, when I had been really quite confident about my ability to treat people with respect. The importance of allowing sufficient time for social interaction before 'getting down to business' was one of those unwritten rules of African culture, which the student knew and practised. And he would never have thought

to point out to me that I was being rude. I was his teacher, and he treated me with respect and did not criticise. (Personal communication, 2005)

In the same way, practice-based educators must also be able to respond to the values, beliefs and ways of 'being' of learners in the practice setting. While there is not space here to explore the concept of 'cultural competence' in detail, a taxonomy adapted from Lister (1999) is shown in Box 4.1. The bibliography at the end of this chapter includes Lister's critique of the concept along with other reading.

Learning and diversity

In Chapters 5 and 6, we explore the notions of learner-centredness and self-directed learning. Attempts to implement these ideas must take account of the fact that what learners think of as 'learning' and what they see as important or useful in a learning task will be shaped by their sociocultural perspectives. What happens to learners whose identities, beliefs and needs in relation to learning have been shaped by a different cultural context from that in which they find themselves? It is important for practice-based educators

---

Box 4.1. A taxonomy of cultural competence (adapted from Lister, 1999)

Cultural awareness
Ability to describe:

- how beliefs, values and power are shaped by culture;
- how different cultures, subcultures and ethnicities validate different beliefs and values.

Cultural knowledge
Familiarity with broad differences, similarities and inequalities in experience, beliefs, values and practices among various groupings in society.

Cultural understanding
Recognising problems and issues faced by individuals when their values, beliefs and practices are compromised by a dominant culture.

Cultural sensitivity
- Showing regard for another's beliefs, values and practices within a cultural context;
- Showing awareness of how one's own cultural background may be influencing professional practice as an educator.

Cultural competence
Providing practice-based education:

- that respects the values, beliefs and practices of the learner;
- which addresses disadvantages arising from the learner's position in relation to networks of power in the organisation.

to try to understand the tensions created between learners' values, attitudes and needs, and those of the organisation. These might reach a critical point during the early period of a practice placement (Stenglehofen, 1993).

In a review of research into the effects of diversity on learning, Pillay (2002) describes cross-cultural variations in concepts such as learning as a duty, persistence (in the face of boredom), valuing problem-solving, help-seeking, collaboration, memorisation, what counts as knowledge and the differentiation between formal and informal learning. Pillay asks some interesting questions, for example:

- Do individuals learn to apply or learn to understand?
- Does the amount of effort we make to learn depend on our perception of how the learning will reward us?
- Is what counts as knowledge the same for all learners?
- Does learning have the same meaning for all learners?

Pillay (2002) Understanding learner-centredness: does it consider the diverse needs of individuals? *Studies in Continuing Education*, 4(1), 93–102.

EXPLORATORY REFLECTION 4.6

- Examine and account for your own beliefs about knowledge and the learning process. How do they compare with those of your colleagues? (You might find it useful to refer back to your response to Exploratory Reflection 4.1.)
- Look back to the list of learners in Exploratory Reflection 4.4. Consider the extent of diversity within the different groups you work with. Discuss how far the issues raised by Pillay are relevant to your own interactions with learners and/or your colleagues.
- Where would you position yourself in Lister's (1999) taxonomy of cultural competence in terms of your interactions with learners?

Legislation and diversity

Diversity encompasses not only different cultural perspectives but also those influenced by gender or disability. Extensive legislation exists to safeguard the rights of individuals and groups to equality of opportunity, and to prevent discrimination, that is unfavourable treatment based on prejudice (Cortis & Law, 2005). Clearly, it is important that as practice-based educators you are aware of the implications of such legislation. It is even more important that you are true to the spirit of an anticipatory and inclusive approach to planning for practice-based learning. This may mean paying attention to your own or others' developmental needs in advance of the learners' arrival, so that changes are already embedded rather than being ad hoc and reactive. This optimises the learning environment for all individuals and makes it more likely they will be empowered to reach their full potential as learners.

EXPLORATORY REFLECTION 4.7

- How familiar are you with legislation related to diversity in your own practice-setting and locale?
- Look back to Chapter 2 for a summary of relevant documents.
- How 'anticipatory and inclusive' are you in fulfilling your role as a practice-based educator for a range of learners?

Summary

This chapter has shown how the practice-based learning environment can influence the quality of learning relationships. Important points to consider are:

- Clinical practice is a challenging environment for learners, with potential for conflicts of interest and loyalty.
- Engendering mutual trust is crucial to effective facilitation of learning.
- Understanding and appreciation of culture and identity are fundamental to building learning relationships and empowering individuals to reach their potential as learners.

Now complete the portfolio sheet for Chapter 4.

- Check how often you are involved in activities associated with creating an optimal environment for learning.
- Consider what evidence you have of your ability to fulfil ACCREDITATION OUTCOME II. Is it sufficient? If not, identify where the gaps lie and how they might be filled.
- Identify your continued developmental needs.
- Reassess your confidence in relation to Chapter 4's learning outcomes, including any personal learning outcomes that you set for yourself.
- Complete your action plan.

Finally, discuss the different ways in which Chapter 4 has helped you to think about your role as a practice-based educator. What reflective purposes has the chapter served for you?

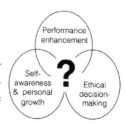

Portfolio Sheet – The Practice-Based Learning Environment

Activities associated with creating a learning environment	Frequency of involvement			Existing evidence for ACCREDITATION OUTCOME II (give details)	Development need?	
	Regularly	Occasionally	Never	*Establish an optimal environment for effective learning*	YES	NO
Monitoring the physical environment in terms of its impact on the learning process.	☐	☐	☐		☐	☐
Building mutual trust between yourself and learners by						
• recognising and minimising potential conflicts of interest or loyalty	☐	☐	☐		☐	☐
• acting as an advocate	☐	☐	☐		☐	☐
• offering supportive challenge	☐	☐	☐		☐	☐
• acting as a sounding board for ideas	☐	☐	☐		☐	☐
• acting as a bridge towards new understanding.	☐	☐	☐		☐	☐
Reflecting with others on issues of culture, identity and diversity that relate to your relationship with learners.	☐	☐	☐		☐	☐
Responding to the social practices and behaviours of others in ways that foster cultural competence in the learning environment.	☐	☐	☐		☐	☐

Sufficient evidence? YES ☐ NO ☐

Chapter 4's Learning Outcomes

	I am confident I can do this	I am not sure I can do this
1. Analyse a range of healthcare settings in terms of the advantages and disadvantages they offer to learners and practice-based educators.	☐	☐
2. Identify and account for specific conflicts of interest you face as an educator and practitioner and analyse their potential impact on your relationship with learners.	☐	☐
3. Evaluate your effectiveness in building trusting relationships with learners in the practice setting.	☐	☐
4. Demonstrate your understanding of the effect of individual differences and needs on learners' and educators' beliefs about the learning process.	☐	☐
5. Identify aspects of legislation relevant to diversity and equal opportunities in learning and education.	☐	☐

Personal learning outcomes for Chapter 4

Confident	Not sure
☐	☐

ACTION PLAN

Bibliography

Brookfield S (1986) *Understanding and Facilitating Adult Learning*. Milton Keynes: Open University Press.

Brookfield S (1990) *The Skilled Teacher*. San Francisco: Jossey-Bass.

Coeling HV, Simms LM (1993) Facilitating innovation at the nursing unit level through cultural assessment, Part 1: How to keep management ideas from falling on deaf ears. *Journal of Nursing Administration*, 23(4), 46–53.

*Cortis J, Law IJ (2005) Anti-racist innovation and nurse education. *Nurse Education Today*, 25(3), 204–213.

Daloz L (1999) *Mentor: Guiding the Journey of Adult Learners*, San Francisco: Jossey-Bass.

*Dunn SV, Hansford B (1997) Undergraduate nursing students' perceptions of their clinical learning environment. *Journal of Advanced Nursing*, 25, 1299–1306.

Hargie O (ed.) (1991) *A Handbook of Communication Skills*. London: Routledge.

Helman CG (1994) *Culture, Health and Illness: An Introduction for Health Professionals*. Oxford: Butterworth-Heinemann.

Heron J (1993) *Group Facilitation: Theories and Models for Practice*. London: Kogan Page.

Hilton R, Morris J (2001) Student placement: is there evidence supporting team skill development in clinical practice settings? *Journal of Interprofessional Care*, 15(2), 171–183.

*Howe A (2001) Patient-centred medicine through student-centred teaching: a student perspective on the key impacts of community-based learning in undergraduate medical education. *Medical Education*, 35(7), 1365–2923.

Hughes C (1999) Facilitation in context. *Studies in Continuing Education*, 21(1), 21–43.

Ilott I, Murphy R (1999) *Success and Failure in Professional Education: Assessing the Evidence*. London: Whurr Publishers.

**Jenkins R (1999) Ethnicity etcetera. Social anthropological points of view. In Bulmer M, Solomos J (eds), *Ethnic and Racial Studies Today*, London and New York: Routledge.

*Kidd W (2002) *Culture and Identity*. Hampshire: Palgrave Macmillan, Chapter 2.

Lickman P, Simms L, Greene C (1993) Learning environment: the catalyst for work excitement. *The Journal of Continuing Education in Nursing*, 24(5), 211–216.

*Lister P (1999) A taxonomy for developing cultural competence. *Nurse Education Today*, 19(4), 313–318.

Maslow A (1954) *Motivation and Personality*. New York: Harper and Row.

†Pillay H (2002) Understanding learner-centredness: does it consider the diverse needs of individuals? *Studies in Continuing Education*, 4(1), 93–102.

Simms LM, Erbin-Roesemann M, Darga A, Coeling H (1990) Breaking the burnout barrier. Resurrecting the work excitement in nursing. *Nursing Economics*, May–June, 177–187.

Stenglehofen J (1993) *Teaching Students in Clinical Settings*. London: Chapman & Hall.

Titchen A (2000) *Professional Craft Knowledge in Patient-Centred Nursing and the Facilitation of its Development.* Kidlington: Ashdale Press.

Williams R (1983) *Key Words: A Vocabulary of Culture and Society,* London: Fontana.

Further reading

*Aronson KR, Venable R, Sieveking N, Miller B (2005) Teaching intercultural awareness to first-year medical students via experiential exercises. *Intercultural Education,* 16(1), 15–24.

*Burnard P (2005) Issues in helping students from other cultures. *Nurse Education Today,* 25(3), 176–180.

Department of Health (2005) Equality and diversity, <http://www.dh.gov.uk/PolicyAndGuidance/HumanResourcesAndTraining/ModelEmployer/EqualityAndDiversity/fs/en> (accessed 4 August 2005).

Larty EY (1997) *In Living Colour. An Intercultural Approach to Pastoral Care and Counselling.* London: Cassell.

**Milner HR (2003) Reflection, racial competence, and critical pedagogy: how do we prepare pre-service teachers to pose tough questions? *Race, Ethnicity and Education,* 6(2), 193–208.

**Trueba E, Takaki R, Muñoz VI, Nieto S (1997) Ethnicity and education forum: what difference does difference make? *Harvard Educational Review,* 67(2), 169–187.

** Suitable for readers who wish to examine concepts at a more detailed or advanced level.
* Suitable for readers looking for something to stimulate ideas in a straightforward way.
† Included in the chapter as suggested reading.

5 LEARNING THEORIES

Introduction In this chapter, we explore how and why adults learn, and introduce some key aspects of learning theory. We encourage you to explore the relevance of learning theories to the process of practice-based learning.

PREPARATORY REFLECTION Working through this chapter should enable you to achieve the learning outcomes listed below. Before continuing, consider how confident you feel now in relation to these outcomes and tick the appropriate box beside each one. Are there any personal learning outcomes you would like to add to the list?

Learning outcomes

	I am confident I can do this	I am not sure I can do this
1. Describe and discuss the characteristics associated with adult learners.	☐	☐
2. Explain the key elements of four related approaches to learning theory.	☐	☐
3. Understand the process of experiential learning and the type of knowledge to which it leads.	☐	☐

	I am confident I can do this	I am not sure I can do this
4. List the skills necessary to engage in effective self-directed learning.	☐	☐
5. Distinguish between 'cooperation' and 'collaboration' in learning.	☐	☐
6. Explain how individual differences in learning style and approach to learning may influence learning outcomes.	☐	☐
7. Use an understanding of learning theory to motivate learners to achieve 'deep' and lasting learning.	☐	☐

Think about any personal outcomes that you would like to add to this list and make a note of them.

Why bother with learning theories?

Why do practice-based educators need to know about learning theories? The answer is two-fold. First of all, learning theories make up an important part of the evidence base for your practice as an educator. Evidence-based clinical practice involves using the best evidence available, in partnership with patients, to decide upon the option most appropriate to their needs. As an effective educator, you should be able to demonstrate how you employ evidence-based methods in your partnership with learners in the practice-based setting. Being able to reflect on your own learning experiences and integrate learning theory into your thinking should help you relate more closely to the needs of the learners you facilitate.

Secondly, as Brookfield (1998) explains, being aware of theory helps practitioners realise that what might seem like signs of their own personal inadequacies as educators can often be interpreted as inevitable consequences of a host of other factors. Not everyone learns in the same way; what counts as 'learning' means different things to different people; individuals differ in their expectations and their readiness to learn in different areas of practice. Being able to draw on learning theory to help explain the impact of such individual differences on learning outcomes prevents educators falling victim to the belief that they are personally responsible for everything that happens during the learning encounter.

EXPLORATORY REFLECTION 5.1

Think about a CPD experience, for example a post-registration course or postgraduate module, directly applicable to your personal-development needs, that you would like to undertake in the future.

- Identify the course/module so that this activity has direct relevance to your own CPD planning.
- State explicitly:
  - o why you want to undertake the course/module;
  - o what you feel you will bring to the learning experience;
  - o what you hope to gain from the learning experience.
- Describe how you will prepare yourself prior to starting the course/module.
- Describe how you will approach the learning activities/assignments.
- State which learning activities/assignments you are especially looking forward to.

Keep your responses close to hand as you work through this chapter.

Adults as learners   Individuals embarking on higher and professional education are all adult learners. To a greater or lesser extent, all of them bring their own past experience of the learning and teaching process. This experience will have influenced and shaped their attitudes and approaches to any new learning challenge. Knowles (1983, 1996), an influential writer on adult learning, suggests that there is an important difference in the ways children and adults regard their experiences.

To a child, experience is an external event rather than an integral part of him- or herself. Asked who they are, children are likely to reply in terms of who their parents are, who their brothers and sisters are, where they live and what school they attend. Self-identity is largely derived from external sources.

Adults define who they are, establish their self-identity, in terms of their accumulated and unique experiences. Asked who they are, adults are likely to define themselves in terms of their occupation, work history, where they have travelled, what education and experience have enabled them to do and what their achievements have been. An adult is what he or she has done.

> If in an educational situation an adult's experience is ignored, not valued, not made use of, it is not just the experience that is being rejected, it is the person.
> (Knowles, 1983, p. 61)

Assumptions about adult learners

Relating new learning to existing experience is a key feature of Knowles' four primary assumptions about adult learners.

1. Adults see themselves as self-directing and responsible.
2. They possess an accumulation of experience which provides a resource for their own learning and that of others.

3. Adults are motivated to learn when they perceive the activity as being directly related to their own activities and when they perceive a need to know something.
4. Their interests tend to focus on problem-solving rather than abstract content or theory.

EXPLORATORY REFLECTION 5.2

- What are your thoughts about the characteristics of adult learners described by Knowles? Do you think they are exclusive to adults – could they also apply to the way children and adolescents learn? Do they apply to *all* adult learners?
- Return to the notes you made during Exploratory Reflection 5.1. Are any of the characteristics Knowles identifies evident in your account of how you intend to approach your planned learning experience?

Stages of learner development

More recent commentators on Knowles' assumptions portray them as aspirational – an ideal for learners and educators to strive towards (Kember *et al.*, 2003). It has become more common to see them as lying at the higher end of a continuum of learner development, from needing highly structured, teacher-centred experiences to seeking more collaborative, learner-centred experiences. In this view, some adult learners may never display the characteristics attributed to them by Knowles.

Developmental psychology has provided some useful frameworks for describing how learners progress towards more complex ways of thinking and understanding. One that has stood the test of time is that of Perry (1970). According to Perry, learners progress from a 'dualist position', in which everything is either 'right' or 'wrong', to one in which they can recognise and accept different points of view (Box 5.1).

EXPLORATORY REFLECTION 5.3

- Think about your own experiences as a learner in terms of Perry's developmental framework, particularly experiences that have occurred more recently.
- Are there any occasions when you have 'regressed' temporarily to a dualist or pluralist perspective when faced with an unfamiliar or particularly challenging learning situation?

Box 5.1. Stages of learning development

DUALISM

Learners recognise only two aspects of a situation – 'right' or 'wrong'. Each question has only one correct answer. The educator has this answer and learners should not differ from this; those who do so are wrong. Learners desperately want to find out which answers the educator prefers. Their need for security is satisfied by educators who transmit their own knowledge directly to the learners.

PLURALISM

From this position learners realise that there may be more than one, or more than only a right or wrong answer and that even authorities may have different opinions. This confuses learners because they do not know what to believe. On the other hand, they mature to the level of needing to express their own opinions as well.

RELATIVISM

Here Perry points out that everyone possesses only a limited vision of reality. No one has perfect perspective. Learners feel they ought not to criticise another who expresses a different opinion from their own. This position differs from 'pluralism' in that learners accept the complexity of reality, rather than simply becoming confused. They experience freedom to differ from other people and from themselves.

COMMITMENT

In this phase learners come to feel the need to widen their vision and draw their own conclusions. This represents real security for learners, who now feel independent and no longer threatened by others' opinions and viewpoints.

(Adapted from Perry, 1970)

Adult learning and other approaches to learning theory
As well as developmental theory, which emphasises individual differences within general stages or levels of learning development, the notion of 'adult learning', or andragogy, spans several broad categories or approaches to learning theory. For example:

- Behaviourism emphasises the value of active 'learning by doing' rather than passive learning. It values feedback as a means to motivate learners and reinforce desirable learning behaviour.
- Cognitive psychology emphasises the need for learners to contextualise new information and enables learners to make links with what they know already.
- A humanistic approach emphasises the need for relevance and personal choice, tailoring learning experiences to the learner's own purposes and goals.

Below are two articles that expand on some of the learning
theories mentioned above.

Coulter (1990) A review of two theories of learning and
their application in the practice of nurse education. *Nurse
Education Today*, 10, 333–338.

Hulse (1992) Learning theories: something for everyone. *Radiologic Technology*, 63(3), 198–202.

- Select one that stimulates your interest and read it carefully.
- How relevant would the concepts outlined in the article be to your planned
  learning experience in Exploratory Reflection 5.1?
- In your opinion, how relevant are the concepts to practice-based learning
  in general?

Types of learning

It should be apparent from this discussion that a
number of different types of learning used in the
practice setting espouse the principles of adult learning (Fry *et al.*, 2003).
Experiential learning, self-directed learning and collaborative learning are
three we will look at in detail here. Others are introduced in subsequent
chapters, for example peer learning and problem-based learning.

Experiential learning

> ... in experiential learning the learner is directly involved with the realities being
> studied. This can be contrasted with learning which is only read, heard or written
> about, but where the reality of practice is never brought into the learning pro-
> cess ... not merely theory but practice, not simply observing but doing. (Hull &
> Redfern, 1996, p. 25)

In Chapter 1, we introduced a cycle of reflection based on work by Kolb
(1984). Kolb's learning cycle (Figure 5.1) defines the basic principles of experiential learning, which have subsequently been adapted by writers on reflective
practice. The original cycle involves four elements of activity.

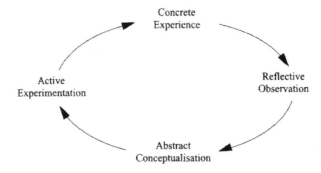

Figure 5.1. Kolb's experiential learning cycle (adapted from Kolb, 1984).

1. Concrete experience – being fully involved in an experience;
2. Reflective observation – thinking critically about what you have done or been involved in;
3. Abstract conceptualisation – making connections between the new experience and other previous experiences, looking for patterns and starting to theorise about what these might be;
4. Active experimentation – testing out your new ideas in the real world, bringing your theory and practice together.

Simply having experience is not the same thing as learning from it. Therefore, movement through all four stages is necessary for effective learning to occur.

Knowledge and experiential learning

Underlying the theory of experiential learning is the belief that knowledge is acquired most effectively not in formal settings, that is removed from reality, but in the informal, everyday context in which it was first created. Lave and Wenger (1991) describe this as situated cognition. This idea of learning in relation to a particular context is at the heart of experiential learning. Knowledge acquired through experiential learning is termed 'professional knowledge' (Eraut, 1994). However, acquiring professional knowledge in context is one thing; being able to describe and explain it is another. It is more difficult to explain knowledge you have gained through your own experience than received knowledge acquired from lectures, research papers or textbooks (formal learning). Classically, this has been described as 'knowing more than we can say' (Polanyi, 1958). We all realise this as soon as we start to reflect seriously upon our own practice!

> Adso: And so, if I understand you correctly, you act and you know why you act, but you don't know [how] you know that you know what you do?
>
> William: Perhaps that's it. In any case, this tells you why I feel so uncertain of my truth even if I believe in it. (Adapted from Eco, 1984, p. 207)

This quotation from Eco's novel illustrates aptly how the difficulty of explaining knowledge gained through experience can cause us to be uncertain about the foundations of our practice as clinicians or educators.

EXPLORATORY REFLECTION 5.4

• Think of some occasions when you have been asked the question 'How do you know that?' by a learner. Think of occasions when your response has involved:

  o repeating received knowledge (perhaps even referring the learner to the
    same text);
  o explaining clearly how your own experience helped you to create a par-
    ticular piece of professional knowledge and act in response to it.
- Which response came most easily to you? To what extent did you, consciously or unconsciously, use Kolb's experiential learning cycle as a framework for describing to the learner how your own experience resulted in
  professional rather than received knowledge?
- What sort(s) of knowledge are you expecting to acquire during the planned
  learning experience you identified in Exploratory Reflection 5.1?

Self-directed learning

It is important to acknowledge that learning and developmental programmes
for healthcare professionals at any level cannot furnish learners with everything they are going to need for continuing practice. Although this might
seem obvious, all too often professional educators, in both higher education
and clinical practice, overload learners with information in an attempt to
bring them up to their own level of competence and skill. Practitioners with
a wealth of practice-based experience sometimes find it difficult to remember
what it was like to function professionally at a lower level of expertise. They
find it hard to relate to the needs of learners, and their expectations may be
inappropriate or unrealistic. They may attempt to compensate for learners'
lack of knowledge by attempting constantly to top up their knowledge base.
Conversely, the demands and constraints of practice make it difficult and
inappropriate for practice-based educators to focus excessively on the needs
of learners.

Self-directed learning skills

By casting them only as passive recipients of information, educators can compromise learners' personal and professional development. Unless learners are
actively involved in seeking knowledge and understanding, and processing
information, there are no guarantees that, because the teacher has taught,
the learner has learnt! Active, self-directed learning falls within the realm
of cognitive psychology, in particular constructivist theory. This is concerned
with how learners construct new knowledge and understanding actively for
themselves, rather than being dependent upon teachers or existing published
knowledge (Seabrook, 2000; Brockett & Hiemstra, 1991). This is one of the
most powerful arguments for encouraging self-directed learning behaviours
in the practice setting. These behaviours include being able to:

a. ask critical questions and analyse problems;
b. define what needs to be learnt and be able to access relevant resources;

c. adopt appropriate learning strategies;
d. be open-minded to other points of view;
e. cope with ambiguity, uncertainty and change;
f. understand your own limitations as a learner and practitioner;
g. observe and use experts as models for improving your own performance;
h. assess your own performance and make plans for improvement;
i. accept that facing setbacks and overcoming difficulties are essential parts of the learning process;
j. remain positive and self-motivating.

This list of skills demonstrates three fundamental elements of self-directed learning.

1. It is an ability to acquire knowledge and skills with minimal assistance from others, for example by setting goals, identifying and using resources.
2. It involves an internal change of perspective on the nature of knowledge, learning and learning relationships.
3. It requires a degree of self-awareness and courage.

> ... some adults are incapable of engaging in self-directed learning because they lack independence, confidence or resources. Not all adults prefer the self-directed option, and even adults who practise self-directed learning also engage in more formal ... teacher directed courses. (Lowry, 1989)

EXPLORATORY REFLECTION 5.5

The most successful [learners] are rarely the cleverest, but are those who feel motivated ... and who persist. Ultimately, all [health professionals] have to rely on their own self-directed learning. Developing these skills early will help ensure success in later careers. (Seabrook, 2000, p. 349)

- Discuss with colleagues the extent to which you
  o use the self-directed learning skills listed above in your own learning;
  o actively encourage such skills in the learners with whom you work.
- To what extent will you need to use self-directed learning skills during the planned learning experience you identified in Exploratory Reflection 5.1?
- Which of the skills a–j above will be most relevant?

Collaborative learning

Focusing only on how individuals set about constructing knowledge for themselves (cognitive constructivism) is limited because it does not take into account how people learn from each other. Therefore, another aspect of constructivist theory – social constructivism – is of equal importance in professional learning.

Constructivism not only identifies the importance of collaborative and active learning. Learning . . . is more effective when learners have opportunities to interact with others and the environment. (Duncombe & Armour, 2004, p. 149)

(Notice that the idea of 'interaction with the environment' takes us back to Lave and Wenger's (1991) notion of 'situated cognition' mentioned earlier in this chapter.)

In Chapter 6, we consider ways in which practice-based educators can put the theory of social constructivism into practice by fostering a collaborative approach to learning. At this point it might be helpful to forestall some possible confusion over terminology by making a distinction between 'collaboration' and 'cooperation'.

Recognizing the difference between cooperation and collaboration is an essential part of the process of enabling [learners] to learn together by engaging in reflective, collaborative, problem-solving activities. (Duncombe & Armour, 2004, p. 146)

Cooperation involves learners working together at the level of giving advice and help, sharing resources, swapping ideas or techniques. It does not involve exploring problems at a deeper level.

Collaboration involves a genuine desire and active interest in identifying and solving problems jointly. Inherent in this approach is commitment to assisting fellow learners, as far as possible, to achieve their own learning goals as well as goals shared by the group.

When planning practice-based learning activities, it can be useful to think of cooperation and collaboration as points on a continuum, and we provide an opportunity for you to relate some activities to this continuum in Chapter 6.

Control of the learning process

As we pointed out at the start of this chapter, achieving 'adulthood' is not synonymous with acquiring the skills of 'adult learning'. Effective adult learning depends in large measure on the acceptance of responsibility and a degree of control by learners over their own learning experiences. However, not all learners are ready or able to take responsibility, and not all educators are fully prepared to share control. A partnership approach to sharing control helps in cultivating and practising the skills of adult learning (Nolan & Nolan, 1997; Slevin & Lavery, 1991). Figure 5.2 illustrates how shared control between the learner and the practice-based educator might be achieved.

This partnership model demonstrates what Hesketh and Laidlaw (2002) describe as the FAIR principles for effective practice as a facilitator of self-directed learning.

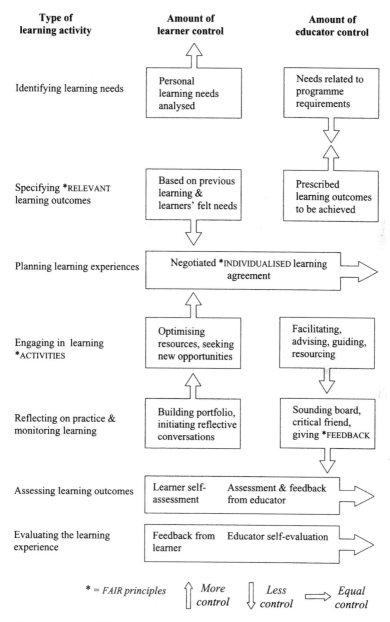

Figure 5.2. A partnership approach to control of the learning process.

- Constructive and frequent *Feedback throughout, not just at the end of, practice-based learning experiences encourages learners to self-assess and motivates them to address their deficiencies and learning needs. (For further detail on 'feedback', see Chapters 6 and 7.)
- Providing a range of practice-based *Activities that promote self-directed and collaborative learning, such as problem-based learning, peer learning, group project work and action-learning sets, encourages learners to develop into active rather than passive learners. (These activities are explored in Chapter 6.)
- An *Individualised approach means learning can cater for the learner's perceived needs, including preferred style, method and pace of learning in the practice setting. Assisting learners to draw up learning agreements relating to the essential components of the practice-based learning experience gives direction to both the learning process and outcomes, but the needs, wishes and individuality of learners are integrated and respected. (For further detail on learning agreements, see Chapter 6.)
- *Relevance enhances the likelihood of learning outcomes being achieved and enhances motivation by ensuring learning experiences are meaningful to the learner's aspirations, goals and practice context.

Learning styles

Learners approach the challenge of taking responsibility for their own learning in different ways. We all have different learning styles that suit us as individuals. They reflect the way in which we approach study as well as the way we think. Learning styles are related to personality and have nothing to do with intelligence. Honey and Mumford (2000a) have developed a classification of learning styles that is one of the most widely used. Based on Kolb's (1984) learning cycle, it describes four groups of characteristics associated with Activists, Reflectors, Theorists and Pragmatists (Table 5.1).

An awareness of learners' preferred learning styles makes it easier for practice-based educators, as well as learners themselves, to identify those learning opportunities from which they are likely to benefit most. Understanding how individuals respond in learning situations can also help educators adapt their style of communication and facilitation in order to optimise learning. The learning styles of learners and practice-based educators will often differ; therefore, it is important that both are encouraged to develop other styles to avoid tension and enable them to utilise all four stages of the learning cycle (Klasen & Clutterbuck 2002).

EXPLORATORY REFLECTION 5.6

Read the description and summaries of Honey and Mumford's learning styles (Table 5.1).

Table 5.1. Characteristics associated with four different learning styles

Activists
- engage fully, without bias, in new experiences
- enjoy the here and now
- open-minded, not sceptical
- enthusiastic about anything new
- dash in where angels fear to tread
- like brainstorming problems
- are bored by implementation and long-term consolidation
- are gregarious and involve themselves with others
- seek to centre all the activities around themselves

Summary
- Positive about learning, make good use of opportunities
- Dislike planning and preparation
- Not keen to reflect on learning
- Can dominate situations because of their enthusiasm

Reflectors
- like to stand back to ponder experiences, thoughtful
- observe from a variety of perspectives
- collect data, think things through before reaching conclusions
- tend to postpone reaching conclusions
- are cautious, leave no stone unturned
- prefer to take a back seat in meetings and discussions
- enjoy observing people in action
- listen to others
- adopt a low profile
- have a slightly distant, tolerant, unruffled air

Summary
- Don't attempt to dominate
- Plan and prepare well
- Good at drawing out the learning from situations
- May be reluctant to take risks
- Don't always grasp opportunities when they arise

Theorists
- integrate observations into complex, logical theories
- think problems through step by step
- assimilate disparate facts into a cohesive whole
- tend to be perfectionists
- like to analyse
- feel uncomfortable with subjective judgements
- tend to be detached, analytical and rational

Summary
- Excellent at identifying underlying causes and relationships
- Set high standards
- May complicate issues and not accept the obvious, hence fail to get action
- Less interested in emotions and feelings

Pragmatists
- like to try out ideas, theories and techniques in the 'real world'
- search out new ideas
- like to experiment
- like to get on with things and act quickly
- tend to be impatient with lengthy, open-ended discussion
- are essentially practical, like making practical decisions
- tend to respond to problems and opportunities as a challenge

Summary
- Positive and anticipate improvement
- Like 'relevant' learning and practical solutions
- Dislike theories and concepts
- May not encourage long-term solutions
- May look for solutions that fit in with the status quo

(Adapted from Honey & Mumford, 2000a, 2000b; and Klasen & Clutterbuck, 2002)

- Which style, or combination of styles, do you associate with yourself?
- How do you think this influences the way you behave as a practice-based educator?
- Compare your preferred style(s) with that of any learners you are currently working with.
- Discuss with them any recent learning situations that demonstrate your compatibility or incompatibility in terms of learning style.
- Explore ways in which you might both utilise a wider range of learning styles to enhance the learning experience and encourage self-directed learning.

Transfer of learning

Earlier in this chapter, we linked experiential learning to the idea that knowledge is acquired most effectively not in formal settings removed from reality but in the informal, everyday context in which it was first created. Check back to remind yourself of the terms used to describe this. However, there are dangers inherent in linking learning too tightly to context.

> A particular danger of the work-based curriculum is the danger of trapping learners' understanding within their own work setting. That is, learners may well learn how to improve their immediate practice, but, constrained to that environment they will be unable to move beyond it ... How can we ensure [they] can apply their learning in situations other than the ones in which they developed it? (Boud & Solomon, 2001, p. 40)

We identified earlier that one of the skills of the self-directed learner is being able to transfer or apply learning across a range of situations, which may have some similarities but which may also be widely dissimilar – and this calls for courage and the ability to deal with uncertainty. Learners must be able to recognise and separate out knowledge learnt in one context to make it available for use in a new situation. How well this is achieved depends on the level at which the original learning was approached.

Levels of processing

Very different approaches to completing the learning task have been described (Marton & Saljo, 1984). There is a direct relationship between these approaches (levels of processing) and the quality of learning outcomes.

Deep levels of processing are thought to lead to the attainment of concepts. Concepts enable us to make sense of a complex array or material and information. The formation and utilisation of concepts are important features of healthcare practice that go beyond simply using knowledge as soon as it is acquired. Strategies associated with this approach involve:

- identifying main ideas, key themes or underlying principles;
- reorganising and synthesising information in light of previous knowledge;
- viewing information from more than one perspective through collaboration with others.

Such strategies enable learners to develop an active awareness of their own learning processes (metacognition – which is the knowledge concerning your own thoughts and the factors that influence your thinking, literally 'thinking about thinking') and to maintain their understanding for longer periods. They are fundamental to recognising the relevance of existing knowledge in any new and unfamiliar practice situations in the future.

Superficial approaches to processing encourage rote learning and memorisation and cause knowledge to remain context-bound and more difficult to recognise and apply in new situations. The strategy associated with this approach is to exert the minimum amount of time and effort necessary to complete the learning task.

Learning intention The use of any particular strategy does not necessarily indicate that a learner is committed to either a deep or superficial approach. A more reliable indication is the purpose or intention of the learner in using strategies (Chalmers & Fuller, 1996). Thus, memorising details may only be used as a preliminary to help in working with ideas at a deeper level. Also in reality, even when we might wish otherwise, sometimes the pressures of the practice setting can cause learners to cut corners and fail to process their learning thoroughly (Boud & Solomon, 2001).

The following comments from some undergraduate health professionals typify the two approaches to learning described above. They also illustrate how a learner's approach can change with increasing commitment to a career path and the associated increase in motivation.

I tried to picture the processes as I went along – to see it all working. I spent time relating the text to my diagrams.

At the end of each section, I ensured that new material was put into perspective and that my newfound knowledge 'fitted in' . . . finally structure and function had become very much as one in the overall picture.

I read the book and took notes – there seemed a lot to read and remember.

I read through the chapter – bits I had done at A level. I skipped through very quickly. It was hard to remember without writing simple notes.

I'm taking more notice, showing more interest. I take longer, I follow up references . . . I try to learn, not just read [because] I've been told to.

On this course, my approach is different because this is the real thing as far as careers are concerned. Basically, my approach is far more serious and perhaps, hopefully, more mature.

EXPLORATORY REFLECTION 5.7

- Return to your planned learning experience in Exploratory Reflection 5.1. Make a judgement about the likely quality of your learning outcome based on what you have learnt about learning styles, approaches and strategies.
- Make a similar judgement about any learners with whom you are working. Most importantly, think about how the learners' efforts and endeavours are being supported. Are they allowed enough space to process their learning thoroughly?

At the start of this chapter, we identified four broad approaches to learning theory: 'behaviourism', 'cognitive psychology', 'developmental' and 'humanistic'. From your reading you will have discovered that these approaches are not mutually exclusive but have areas of overlap. Being aware of theories underlying learning will help you to understand better the variations in behaviour and response you see in learners you work with, as well as in your own learning. Also, as Figure 5.3 illustrates, it will enable you to decide how best to assist learners to achieve deep, lasting learning and maximise the learning potential of the practice-based setting.

Summary

This chapter has explored the value of learning theories to practice-based educators. Important points to consider are:

- Understanding how people learn is a valuable basis for practice-based educators to provide effective facilitation for learners.
- Theories about how people learn are closely interrelated.
- Learners and educators vary in their readiness and ability to use the skills and strategies associated with adult learning.
- Developing the skills of self-directed learning and collaborative learning is fundamental to achieving the status of a competent, reflective, autonomous healthcare practitioner.

Now complete the portfolio sheet for Chapter 5.

- Check how often you use aspects of learning theory to optimise your effectiveness as a practice-based educator.
- Consider what evidence you have of your ability to fulfil ACCREDITATION OUTCOME III. Is it sufficient? If not, identify where the gaps lie and how they might be filled.
- Identify your continued-development needs.

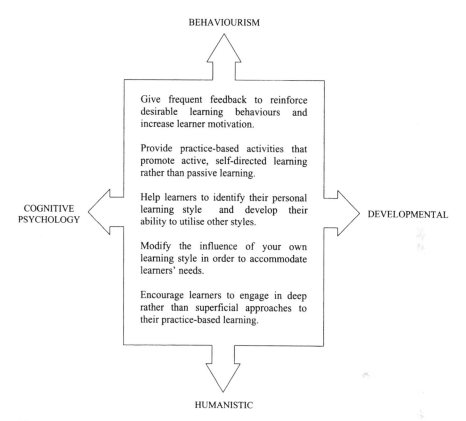

Figure 5.3. Using learning theories to facilitate learning.

- Reassess your confidence in relation to Chapter 5's learning outcomes, including any personal learning outcomes you identified for yourself.
- Complete your action plan.

Finally, discuss the different ways in which Chapter 5 has helped you to think about your role as a practice-based educator. What reflective purposes has the chapter served for you?

Portfolio Sheet – Learning Theories

Activities associated with applying learning theory	Frequency of use — Regularly	Occasionally	Never	Existing evidence for ACCREDITATION OUTCOME III (give details)	Development need? YES	NO
				Apply learning theories that are appropriate for adult and professional learners		
Giving frequent feedback to reinforce desirable learning behaviours and increase learner motivation.	☐	☐	☐		☐	☐
Providing practice-based activities that promote active, self-directed learning rather than passive learning.	☐	☐	☐		☐	☐
Providing opportunities for learners to engage in collaborative learning with others.	☐	☐	☐		☐	☐
Helping learners identify their personal learning style and developing their ability to utilise other styles.	☐	☐	☐		☐	☐
Modifying the influence of your own learning style in order to accommodate learners' needs.	☐	☐	☐		☐	☐
Encouraging learners to engage in deep rather than superficial approaches to their practice-based learning.	☐	☐	☐		☐	☐
Sharing responsibility and control of the learning process with learners.	☐	☐	☐		☐	☐

Sufficient evidence? YES ☐ NO ☐

Chapter 5's Learning Outcomes

	I am confident I can do this	I am not sure I can do this
1. Describe and discuss the characteristics associated with adult learners.	☐	☐
2. Explain the key elements of four related approaches to learning theory.	☐	☐
3. Understand the process of experiential learning and the type of knowledge to which it leads.	☐	☐
4. List the skills necessary to engage in effective self-directed learning.	☐	☐
5. Distinguish between 'cooperation' and 'collaboration' in learning.	☐	☐
6. Explain how individual differences in learning style and approach to learning may influence learning outcomes.	☐	☐
7. Use an understanding of learning theory to motivate learners to achieve 'deep' and lasting learning.	☐	☐

Personal learning outcomes for Chapter 5

	Confident	Not sure
	☐	☐

ACTION PLAN

Bibliography

Boud D, Solomon N (eds) (2001) *Work-Based Learning: A New Higher Education?* Buckingham: Society for Research into Higher Education and Open University Press.

Brockett RG, Hiemstra R (1991) *Self-direction in Adult Learning: Perspectives on Theory, Research and Practice.* New York: Routledge.

Brookfield S (1998) Critically reflective practice. *The Journal of Continuing Education in the Health Professions,* 18(4), 197–205.

Chalmers D, Fuller R (1996) *Teaching for Learning at University.* London: Kogan Page.

†Coulter MA (1990) A review of two theories of learning and their application in the practice of nurse education. *Nurse Education Today,* 10, 333–338.

Duncombe R, Armour KM (2004) Collaborative professional learning: from theory to practice. *Journal of In-Service Education,* 30(1), 141–166.

Eco U (1984) *The Name of the Rose.* London: Picador in association with Secker & Warburg.

Eraut M (1994) *Developing Professional Knowledge and Competence.* London: Falmer Press.

Fry H, Ketteridge S, Marshall S (2003) Understanding student learning. In Fry H, Ketteridge S, Marshall S (eds), *A Handbook for Teaching and Learning in Higher Education.* London: Kogan Page.

Hesketh EA, Laidlaw JM (2002) Developing the teaching instinct 3: facilitating learning. *Medical Teacher,* 24(5), 479–482.

*Honey P, Mumford A (2000a) *The Learning Styles Questionnaire: 80-Item Version.* Peter Honey Publications, ISBN: 1902899075.

*Honey P, Mumford A (2000b) *The Learning Styles Helper's Guide.* Peter Honey Publications, ISBN: 1902899105.

Hull C, Redfern L (1996) *Profiles and Portfolios: A Guide for Nurses and Midwives.* London: Macmillan.

†Hulse SF (1992) Learning theories: something for everyone. *Radiologic Technology,* 63(3), 198–202.

Kember D, Jenkins W, Ng KC (2003) Adult students' perceptions of good teaching as a function of their conceptions of learning – part 1: influencing the development of self-determination. *Studies in Continuing Education,* 25(2), 239–251.

Klasen N, Clutterbuck D (2002) *Implementing Mentoring Schemes: A Practical Guide to Successful Programs.* London: Butterworth-Heinemann.

Knowles M (1983) The modern practice of adult education: from pedagogy to andragogy. In Jobling MH, Tight M (eds), *Adult Learning and Education.* London: Croom Helm in association with the Open University.

Knowles M (1996) Andragogy: an emerging technology for adult learning. In Edwards R, Hanson A, Raggett P (eds), *Boundaries of Adult Learning.* London: Routledge.

Kolb DA (1984) *Experiential Learning.* Englewood Cliffs, NJ: Prentice-Hall.

Lave J, Wenger E (1991) *Situated Learning: Legitimate Peripheral Participation.* New York: Cambridge University Press.

Lowry CM (1989) Supporting and facilitating self-directed learning. ERIC Digest No. 93, <http://www.ericdigests.org/pre-9213/self.htm>, accessed 11 August 2005.

Marton F, Saljo R (1984) Approaches to learning. In Marton F, Hounsell D, Entwistle N (eds), *The Experiences of Learning*. Edinburgh: Scottish Academic Press.

Nolan J, Nolan M (1997) Self-directed and student-centred learning in nurse education. *British Journal of Nursing*, 6(2), 103–107.

Perry WG (1970) *Forms of Intellectual and Ethical Development in the College Years*. New York: Holt, Reinhart & Winston.

Polanyi M (1958) *Personal Knowledge*. London: Routledge and Kegan Paul.

Seabrook M (2000) Self-directed learning or DIY education? *Student BMJ*, 8 October.

Slevin OD'A, Lavery MA (1991) Self-directed learning and student supervision. *Nurse Education Today*, 11, 368–377.

Further reading

**Child D (1993) *Psychology and the Teacher*. London: Cassell.

Crandall S (1993) How expert clinical educators teach what they know. *Journal of Continuing Education in the Health Professions*, 13(1), 85–98.

**Kaufman DM, Mann KV, Jennett PA (2000) *Teaching and Learning in Medical Education: How Theory Can Inform Practice*. Edinburgh: Association for the Study of Medical Education.

**Merriam SB (1996) Updating our knowledge of adult learning. *Journal of Continuing Education in the Health Professions*, 16(3), 136–143.

** Suitable for readers who wish to examine concepts at a more detailed or advanced level.
* Suitable for readers looking for something to stimulate ideas in a straightforward way.
† Included in the chapter as suggested reading.

6 FACILITATING LEARNING IN THE PRACTICE SETTING

Introduction   So far we have talked the talk of practice-based learning by examining its context, introducing a selection of relevant learning theories and considering what we mean by reflective learning. However, the main purpose of the book is to enable you to walk the walk as a practice-based educator with increased confidence. Therefore, in this chapter we describe a variety of ways in which you can actually set about the task of facilitating adult learning in the practice setting. The chapter opens with an outline of what we mean by facilitation. Then, because it is the largest chapter in the book, we have made the remainder easier to navigate by dividing it into a flexible facilitation toolkit made up of four sections. You may choose to dip into sections in any order to select methods and ideas that suit your needs.

   Inevitably, our choices are not exhaustive. If you are an experienced educator, you may already use a range of facilitation methods in your own practice setting. You will be able to add items from your own repertoire to the toolkit. Those of you who are new educators may find our suggestions a useful starting point, but ultimately you will adapt them for your own use and develop your own personalised approach.

PREPARATORY REFLECTION

Working through this chapter should enable you to achieve the learning outcomes listed below. Before continuing, consider how confident you feel now in relation to these outcomes and tick the appropriate box beside each one. Are there any personal learning outcomes you would like to add to the list?

Learning outcomes

	I am confident I can do this	I am not sure I can do this
1. Discuss key principles underpinning facilitation of learning in the practice setting.	☐	☐
2. Explain the significance of the relationship between practice-based educator and learner in the facilitation process.	☐	☐
3. Select and justify the use of a range of methods to		
○ plan and structure learning in the practice setting;	☐	☐
○ foster collaboration between peers and teams;	☐	☐
○ promote independence in practice-based learners.	☐	☐
4. Employ appropriate strategies for avoiding and/or resolving problems associated with practice-based learning, facilitation and learning relationships.	☐	☐

(You might find it helpful to look ahead to the portfolio sheet at the end of this chapter, which lists the ideas and methods covered.)

Think about any personal outcomes that you would like to add to this list and make a note of them.

What do we mean by facilitation?

> Facilitation is a technique by which one person makes something easier for others.
> (Rycroft-Malone *et al.*, 2002, p. 177)

Facilitation is about helping and enabling rather than telling and persuading. Any learning experience is a two-way process with opportunities for both educator and learner to facilitate each other in their respective roles. For example, a new practice educator embarking on her/his first practice placement may benefit from the valuable feedback that learners can provide. This mutual process of facilitation stimulates reciprocal dialogue and trust so that both parties can learn from the experience (Ireland, 2003; Alsop & Ryan, 1996). Gilmartin (2001) also suggests that key qualities for the facilitator are an ability to listen actively, possessing an understanding of group dynamics and the ability to make best use of peer-learning opportunities.

EXPLORATORY REFLECTION 6.1   Look back to Chapter 3 to remind yourself of the wide variety of elements that make up the facilitator's role in the practice setting.

As Chapter 3 explains, facilitation encompasses a broad range of purposes. These include providing practical help and support to achieve a specific task or goal and enabling learners to reach their potential by analysing and reflecting on their own attitudes, behaviours and ways of working. These purposes are not mutually exclusive but rather points on a continuum from 'task-focused' to 'holistic' facilitation. As your repertoire or toolkit of facilitation methods builds, you will be able to plot them along this continuum.

What do we want to facilitate?

Unless we are sure what we want to promote in learners, our efforts at facilitation could be misdirected. Therefore it is important to consider the multiplicity of skills and abilities required of learners in preparation for contemporary professional practice.

EXPLORATORY REFLECTION 6.2   With a group of colleagues, ask yourselves the question 'What skills and abilities do we want to facilitate in our learners?' Compare your ideas with our thoughts below.

It will be clear from Figure 6.1 that educators in health care are concerned not only with imperatives of current practice but also with anticipating change and uncertainty that lies ahead. They are concerned not only with enhancing profession-specific skills of individuals but also with fostering those that empower practitioners to work together effectively as teams. With this in

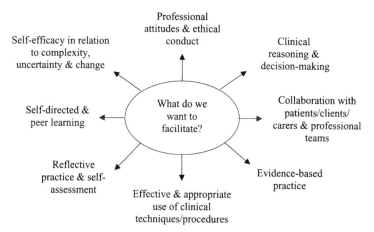

Figure 6.1. Component activities of professional practice.

mind, we can begin to think about processes that facilitate learning in and through practice. Two possible places to start may be your own experiences of being supported by others in role-development activities and/or your experience to date as a practice-based educator.

EXPLORATORY REFLECTION 6.3

Think about your personal experience as either a learner or an educator in the practice setting.

- By what means were you enabled to develop your practice by other people?
- How do *you* fulfil this role in relation to the learning needs of others?

(You might find it helpful to look back to your thoughts in relation to Exploratory Reflection 2.2 in Chapter 2.) Keep a note of your ideas to refer to as you work on constructing your own toolkit.

Principles for the effective facilitation of practice learning

When selecting any facilitation approach, it is worth reviewing the following principles of effective facilitation adapted from the work of Brookfield (1998), who was responsible for 'casting facilitation as a dialogue among equals' (Hughes, 2002, p. 60).

Brookfield's principles draw on and reinforce the key elements of adult learning:

- The decision to learn is the learner's.
- Respect and collaboration between learner and educator are essential for learning to be successful.
- Learning should follow a cycle of activity, which involves the active involvement of learner and educator in the process, followed by reflection and analysis.
- Facilitation should foster self-critical reflection in learners.
- Educators and peers who provide supportive challenge to learners' ideas and interpretations encourage them to explore alternative solutions to practice problems.
- Self-direction should be nurtured in learners by empowering them to take responsibility for their own learning.

These principles highlight the role of praxis in any learning activity. Brookfield (1998) defines 'praxis' as an active cycle which has three key elements:

1. activity involving both learner and educator
2. reflection upon the activity
3. collaborative analysis.

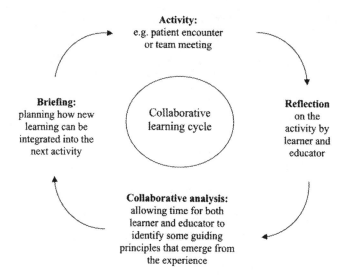

Figure 6.2. Components of a collaborative learning cycle.

Figure 6.2 incorporates the key elements of praxis in a collaborative learning cycle that includes an additional period of briefing before the next activity (Moon, 2000). A comment from a learner in the practice environment illustrates the value of such mutual involvement in the learning process from the initial patient encounter to subsequent exploration and discussion.

> Throughout the placement I have felt that parts of the jigsaw of my knowledge have slotted together through treating patients and then subsequent discussion with my educator about my clinical reasoning. (Postgraduate on specialist practice placement)

Trust between educator and learner

In Chapter 4, we emphasised the importance of a trusting relationship between educators and learners, and, clearly, Brookfield's 'dialogue among equals' must be based on mutual trust.

To fully appreciate the importance of learning relationships built on trust we suggest you read:

Hughes (1999) Facilitation in context. *Studies in Continuing Education*, 21(1), 21–43.

Reflect on the issues raised in the article. How do they relate to your own practice as an educator?

Facilitation and the FAIR principles

The principles of effective practice identified by Brookfield link closely to the FAIR principles for effective practice as a facilitator of self-directed learning (Hesketh & Laidlaw, 2002), which you were introduced to in Chapter 5, namely:

- **F**eedback – that is constructive and frequent.
- **A**ctivities – promoting self-directed learning behaviours.
- **I**ndividualised – approaches to learning.
- **R**elevance – enhancing motivation and ensuring learning outcomes meet the learner's needs.

When selecting approaches from the toolkit or adding your own, it is worth trying to ensure that whenever possible the facilitation approach you choose incorporates each of the FAIR principles in order to promote self-directed learning as effectively as possible.

Stages of practice-based learning and facilitation

Having reviewed some important principles that underpin facilitation of learning, we now consider the stages of learning experienced by learners in the practice setting and consider appropriate methods of facilitation relevant to each stage. Anderson (1988) proposes that the process of facilitating learning in practice settings should enable any learner to move through the following stages:

1. an early stage of direct dependence on the educator who contributes actively towards the learning process;
2. a transitional stage, involving discussion and questioning, in which learning results from increased collaboration between learner and educator, and between learner and peers;
3. an advanced stage of greater independence for the learner involving critical reflection on practice, self-assessment and increased responsibility.

Each stage is worked towards progressively. The pace of the whole process will be determined by individual learner differences, hence negotiating the pace of learning is an important part of the facilitation process. As with any learning experience, the more complex the problems facing learners, the more dependent they become on the educator. Therefore, learners are free to move forwards or backwards along the early–advanced continuum as increasingly challenging situations or unfamiliar contexts arise (Figure 6.3). In Figure 6.4 we have mapped three stages of facilitation activity onto the practice-based learning continuum. In the early stage, this is focused on structuring the learning experience based on learners' needs and readiness. In the transi-

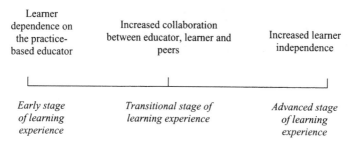

Figure 6.3. Stages of practice-based learning.

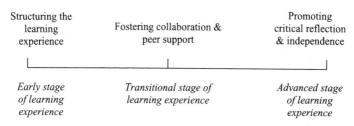

Figure 6.4. Stages of practice-based facilitation.

tional stage, the emphasis is on progressing learners' development by fostering collaboration with educator and peers. In the advanced stage the learners are urged towards greater independence and responsibility through critical reflection on their own and others' practice and through self-assessment.

How can we facilitate learning?

As you might expect, there is a considerable and expanding array of facilitation methods available to practice-based educators, and it probably goes without saying that individual facilitation methods cannot be totally compartmentalised. Inevitably, there is a good deal of overlap. However, we have simplified things by arranging some of the most used methods and ideas into four sections, which together make up our facilitation toolkit.

In Figure 6.5, the toolkit is depicted as a series of drop-down menus similar to those you might work with on your computer. There are four sections or options in the main menu. The first three match the stages of facilitation we identified above (i.e. structuring the learning experience, fostering collaboration and promoting empowerment). Each section has a sub-menu that lists tools or methods that can be used to facilitate learning and development at that particular stage. The fourth section in the main menu – troubleshooting – explores some reasons why things might go wrong in practice-based learning interactions and suggests ideas for dealing with problems.

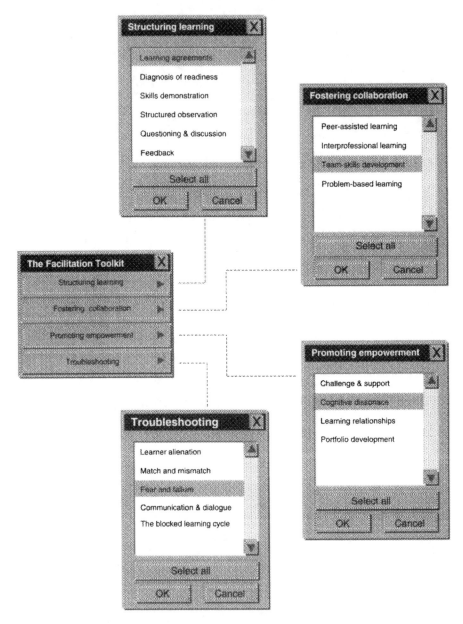

Figure 6.5. The facilitation toolkit.

TOOLKIT SECTION ONE: STRUCTURING LEARNING

Negotiated learning agreements

A learning agreement identifies what a learner wants to learn, how he or she will set about learning it, how and by whom the learning will be assessed and by what standards the performance will be judged. A learning agreement can be an effective facilitation tool for developing skills necessary to engage in self-directed and lifelong learning. Learners are encouraged to reflect on their prior learning, to identify their learning needs and to take an active, rather than passive, part in the learning experience (Anderson *et al.*, 1996). They provide a secure channel through which both parties can raise issues in a constructive way. Therefore, the success of the negotiating process depends on effective communication.

Comments from learners who have used learning agreements highlight the focus and self-direction that they offer.

> I was able to identify areas which I needed to develop. This led to a more structured approach to my learning. (Undergraduate)

> They [learning agreements] indicated to the educator that you were proactive in the learning and enabled you to identify your shortcomings and ask for advice. (Undergraduate)

How does a learning agreement facilitate learning?

In negotiation with their practice-based educator learners are enabled to:

- analyse their personal learning needs and opportunities for further development in relation to the new experience;
- define learning outcomes that show how their learning needs will be fulfilled;
- explore strategies and learning resources that will assist them in achieving their desired learning outcomes;
- plan the most appropriate way in which achievement of the learning outcomes can be assessed.

In Figure 6.6, these elements of the negotiation process are depicted as a cycle, with some useful questions to ask or issues to think about at each point.

Analysing learning needs

Being able to analyse learning needs (one's own and others') is fundamental to the learning process. Learning-needs analysis can take many forms, but ultimately it leads to changes in practice and hence underpins continuing professional development.

1. Analyse learning needs

Questions for the learner:
- What do I already know about this practice area?
- What do I need to know/be able to do?
- Have any previous learning needs been highlighted that I need to share with my educator in this placement?
- What am I looking forward to most?
- What concerns me most?

Questions for the educator:
- What specific opportunities for learning exist in this practice context?
- Which learning needs could be most effectively addressed in this practice setting?
- Can the learning needs be prioritised in terms of *must* be addressed, *should* be addressed, *could* be addressed if time allows?
- Has the learner identified any habitual performance problems that we could help to eliminate in this placement?

4. Planning for assessment *(see Chapter 7)*

- Do the learning outcomes require a quantitative or a qualitative approach to assessment?
- Can the learner take the initiative in deciding on criteria for assessment, for example by describing in her/his own words what good and poor performance would look like?
- Does the assessment pose a stimulating challenge or an anxiety-provoking threat?
- When will the assessment be carried out and who will be involved?

2. Defining learning outcomes

- What levels of *cognitive* skills are represented by the learning outcomes – are they too high/too low/appropriate?
- What categories of *transferable* skills are represented by the learning outcomes?
- Are the learning outcomes assessable in this context?
- Is a means of assessment indicated in the outcome statement?
- Are the learning outcomes achievable in the time available?

3. Identifying strategies & resources

- What human and material resources are available to assist in achieving the learning outcomes?
- Can the learner take the initiative in suggesting suitable learning strategies, for example by discussing her/his personal learning style?
- Is there scope to help the learner experiment with different approaches and develop greater flexibility as a learner?

Figure 6.6. The cycle of negotiation in learning agreements.

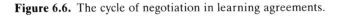

EXPLORATORY REFLECTION 6.4   Practitioners use a variety of formal and informal ways of identifying and analysing their own learning needs as part of their practice (Grant, 2002). Which of the methods listed below have you and/or your colleagues used recently to identify your personal learning needs?

- Clinical audit ☐
- Adverse events ☐
- Risk assessment ☐
- Patient-satisfaction data ☐
- Assessment of competencies ☐
- Peer review ☐
- In-service education ☐
- Self-assessment ☐
- Reflection (diaries, log books, practice reviews) ☐
- Clinical supervision ☐
- Informal conversations ☐
- Semi-structured interviews and focus groups ☐
- Journal articles ☐
- Conferences ☐
- Academic activities ☐

What other means of learning-needs analysis have you used for yourself or for learners that you could add to this list?

Initial learning-needs analysis could be seen as a form of 'semi-structured interview' in which the practice-based educator obtains information about the learner. This is done through use of open questions, such as those in Figure 6.6, around a particular theme (in this case the learner's needs and aspirations in relation to the forthcoming learning experience). Such interviews can often 'yield answers that may reveal uncertainties, conflicts, inconsistencies, unexpected problems, anxieties, fears, and present knowledge base' (Kitchie, 1997, p. 61). As the learning experience proceeds, additional needs may become apparent through some of the other mechanisms listed above. These can be added to the agreement as and when appropriate.

Defining learning outcomes

In the negotiated learning agreement learning outcomes state explicitly what the learner intends to achieve in terms of what he or she knows or can do. They reflect changes in the learner as a result of going through the learning experience.

Learning outcomes should:

- be written in the future tense;
- identify important learning intentions (and requirements);
- be achievable in the time available;
- be assessable in the practice setting;
- use language that
  o makes clear what will be achieved;
  o indicates how achievement could be assessed.

Writing learning outcome statements

In the negotiated learning agreement, learning outcomes always start with the phrase 'I can/will be able to . . .' followed by a descriptive verb. In Box 6.1, cognitive skills are organised into a well-recognised hierarchy of levels of achievement and some appropriate verbs to use are listed. As learners gain experience and engage in more challenging and complex activity in a particular learning context, their learning outcome statements should include some that reflect more sophisticated levels in the hierarchy such as 'synthesis' or 'evaluation'. Transferable skills (Box 6.2) are those we gradually acquire through a whole range of formal and informal learning and life experiences. They are portable skills we carry with us that involve the ability to work with people, things or information across contexts. In Box 6.3 are two less-well-defined taxonomies relating to psychomotor skills (bodily movement triggered by mental activity) and affective skills (external expression of emotion associated with an idea or action).

EXPLORATORY
REFLECTION 6.5

Look at the list of learning outcomes in the sample learning agreement in Figure 6.7. The first outcome is positioned at the lower end of the cognitive skills hierarchy (knowledge and understanding); the second is at a higher level (analysis). Outcome 4 extends the learner to the level of evaluation.

Also notice how the wording of each statement provides a logical link with how it is assessed. For example:

Outcome 1: know what and how clinical investigations are carried out, be able to explain their rationale and interpret results in terms of implications for treatment/management of patients . . . .

- Now try writing some learning outcome statements of your own that reflect
  o different cognitive skill levels;
  o different categories of transferable skills;
  o different levels of psychomotor skill.
- Do your statements give an indication of how they might be assessed?
- With colleagues, discuss the applicability of the affective skills in Box 6.3 to the taxonomy of cultural competence in Chapter 4 (Box 4.1).

Exploring learning strategies and resources

As a practice-based educator, you will probably have a clear idea of human and material resources available to learners in your setting. If you are an experienced educator, you may well have a good idea of the types of learn-

Box 6.1. Useful verbs to use when writing learning outcome statements in a learning agreement: *Cognitive skills domain* (based on Bloom's *Taxonomy*, 1956)

Can you convey what you KNOW?
- Can you provide definitions and descriptions?
- Do you have a sense of what is relevant or not relevant?

Useful verbs: I can/will be able to:

define	choose	match	recognise	describe	list
select	acquire	recall	identify	distinguish	omit

Can you convey what you UNDERSTAND?
- Can you talk about what you know and identify what remains confusing?
- Can you link what you know to other information in your knowledge base?

Useful verbs: I can/will be able to:

explain	discuss	review	clarify	show	translate
rephrase	prepare	illustrate	demonstrate	conclude	restate

Can you APPLY your knowledge?
- Can you recognise different situations/contexts in which to make appropriate use of your knowledge?
- Can you demonstrate your knowledge by teaching it to others?

Useful verbs: I can/will be able to:

demonstrate	predict	generalise	restructure	use	classify
schedule	relate	practise	operate	organise	transfer

Can you ANALYSE what you know?
- Can you break down a particular area of knowledge into parts or forms?
- Can you analyse relationships within and between areas of knowledge?

Useful verbs: I can/will be able to:

compare	examine	distinguish between	hypothesise
experiment	debate	analyse	make assumptions
criticise	question	recognise inconsistencies	contrast

Can you SYNTHESISE what you know?
- Can you make new linkages and combine elements into patterns not clearly seen before?
- Can you use your knowledge to solve complex problems?

Useful verbs: I can/will be able to:

propose	originate	modify	design	combine	construct
create	set up	invent	formulate	conceptualise	devise
develop	produce	elaborate	plan	model	specify

Can you EVALUATE what you know?
- Can you make judgements based on evidence in relation to some set of criteria?
- Can you validate/test your assumptions to build reliability into your knowledge base?

Useful verbs: I can/will be able to:

judge	comment on	validate	assess	appraise	standardise
evaluate	defend	decide	arbitrate	critique	review
discriminate	confirm	measure	decide	advocate	rate/rank

Box 6.2. Useful verbs to use when writing learning outcome statements in a learning agreement: *Transferable skills domain* (based on Allan, 2000)

Can you COLLABORATE and work in TEAMS?
- Do you value collaborative learning and working relationships?
- Do you recognise and acknowledge the value of others' experiences and viewpoints?

Useful verbs: I can/will be able to:

acknowledge	motivate	support	enable	collaborate	respond
facilitate	participate	arbitrate	advocate	encourage	affirm
appreciate	accept	value	share	recognise	cooperate

Are you SELF-DIRECTED and able to ACT INDEPENDENTLY?
- Are you self-motivated and resourceful?
- Can you monitor and assess your own progress?
- Can you reflect upon your own performance and achievements?

Useful verbs: I can/will be able to:

reflect	(re-)evaluate	examine	explore	identify	recognise
search	change	respond	decide	plan	prioritise
access	select	use	compile	develop	learn
find	understand	initiate	assess	organise	improve

Can you THINK CRITICALLY and SOLVE PROBLEMS?
- Can you examine problems from a number of perspectives?
- Can you relate new ideas to existing ideas and frameworks?
- Can you question and challenge viewpoints and ideas constructively on the basis of evidence?
- Can you relate theoretical ideas to practical tasks?

Useful verbs: I can/will be able to:

identify	recognise	formulate	apply	resolve	examine
question	challenge	judge	relate	justify	propose

Can you ACCESS and USE INFORMATION effectively?
- Can you create, store and retrieve information in a variety of forms?
- Can you select, gather and use information acquired from various sources, in effective ways?

Useful verbs: I can/will be able to:

write	select	compile	interpret	analyse	create
search	find	access	synthesise	read	review

Can you COMMUNICATE effectively?
- Can you write in a variety of formats, using appropriate styles for different audiences?
- Can you present material/information graphically and orally in a variety of formats appropriate for different audiences?

Useful verbs: I can/will be able to:

express	explain	argue	question	illustrate	stimulate
articulate	summarise	adapt	design	create	present
use metaphors	draw analogies	perform	involve	inspire	provoke

Box 6.3. Skills in the psychomotor and affective domains

Psychomotor domain: development of physical movement and coordination

Imitate
Observes a skill and tries to replicate it.

Manipulate
No need to observe, able to perform skill according to general instructions.

Precision
Performs skill independently with precision and fluency.

Articulation
Can modify skill or adapt it to fit new situations. Can combine more than one skill in sequence.

Naturalisation
Completes one or more skills with ease and automaticity.

(Dave, 1970)

Affective domain: development of attitudes, beliefs and values

Receiving
Awareness, willingness to hear, listens to others with respect.

Responding
Complies with given expectations, active participation.

Valuing
Overt behaviour consistent with specified values without coercion.

Organisation
Prioritises values, resolves conflicts between them and creates a new value system. Recognises need for balance between freedom and responsible behaviour.

Internalising
Total behaviour is consistent with internalised values.

(Krathwohl *et al.*, 1973)

---

ing strategies that have proved successful for learners in your context in the past. However, it is important to let the learner take the initiative in suggesting how he or she could attempt to achieve the learning outcomes you have negotiated between you. As far as possible, let his or her preferences guide the final choice, unless you feel they place unreasonable demands on you or create problems for your colleagues.

How learners approach the issue of identifying learning strategies and resources can give a useful indication of their existing abilities in relation to transferable skills. This part of the agreement can provide opportunities

NEGOTIATED LEARNING OUTCOMES	LEARNING STRATEGIES & RESOURCES	ASSESSMENT PLAN
I will be able to:	1. CXR teaching session, observation of nurses carrying out spirometry, see a bronchoscopy, use CD ROM and internet facilities in department.	1. Interpret three sets of unseen investigations provided by Jane and discuss implications for patients' treatment/ management.
1. know what and how clinical investigations are carried out, be able to explain their rationale & interpret results in terms of implications for treatment/ management of patients with cystic fibrosis.	2. Observe examination and techniques performed by my educator Jane, & other qualified staff. Use structured observation sheets provided, plus devise my own and add them to the resource folder for other learners.	2. Demonstrate a full examination and/or treatment session observed by Jane, who will use a structured observation sheet and rating scale devised by me to assess my performance.
2. examine patients accurately and efficiently and identify relevant clinical signs and functional problems (and finally know how to use a stethoscope properly!).		3. Carry out audit of my record keeping to track quality of information and patient outcomes.
3. carry out effective interventions based on my assessment findings.	3. Participate in shared treatment sessions with Jane and attend in-service training sessions with other staff. Familiarise myself with British National Formulary & Datasheet Compendium. Visit Pharmacy. Keep a learning log of skills acquired.	4. Feedback on my performance from other members of the team who have had opportunities to observe me on wards or in team meetings will be sought, using a brief feedback sheet devised by me. I will discuss the feedback with Jane.
4. relate the general psychological effects of chronic illness to the specific problems and needs experienced by the people living with cystic fibrosis that I meet during the placement.	4. Initiate contact with other members of the inter- professional team and with carers, and arrange to meet. (Read up in relevant areas and prepare informed questions.) Take active part in weekly team meetings. Access literature on patient partnership and patient satisfaction. Draft relevant criteria and discuss with other members of the team. Prepare a patient feedback sheet on word-processor and get approval to administer it at end of placement.	Collect patient satisfaction data and summarise in short report with descriptive analysis (graph) and content analysis of comments.
5. reflect critically on the placement experience and its demands in order to compare my feelings and performance in this setting with that in previous acute out-patient settings.		5. Prepare 2 reflective statements based on different key incidents that demonstrate how my approach to learning in practice has developed. Discuss with Jane.
	5. Do initial self-assessment against characteristics of reflective/theorist learning style (not me at all!!!). Look at suggestions for expanding learning styles in LS inventory. Discuss ideas with Jane. Keep reflective diary.	

Figure 6.7. An example of a negotiated learning agreement.

to stretch and develop learners in these areas. For example, in relation to Learning Outcome 4 in Figure 6.7, access to resources involves skills of self-direction and collaboration on the part of the learner.

Planning for assessment

In Chapter 7, we discuss the issue of assessment in detail, and in particular the importance of establishing clear links between learning outcome statements and their actual assessment. At this point we offer some general guidelines on planning for an assessment of negotiated learning outcomes.

What you decide to do about assessment depends, to an extent, on the nature of the learning outcomes.

- If the learning outcomes are related to objective performance, you may decide on a quantitative approach, which identifies specific criteria and a minimum standard to be reached.
- If the outcomes are more concerned with subjective feelings or attitudes, you may decide on a qualitative approach, which tries to gain insights or illuminate a particular situation, for example a journal or series of reflective statements.
- You and the learner should cooperate in deciding a method with which you can both cope because, if the outcome is disappointing, you will both need to consider your contribution to the situation.
- Be realistic – don't set standards that only a superhero could achieve!
- Keep it simple and straightforward – create a challenge, not a threat.

EXPLORATORY REFLECTION 6.6

With a group of colleagues, discuss the potential value of negotiated learning agreements in your own professional development as practice-based educators and practitioners.

- What do you consider are some advantages and disadvantages of negotiated learning agreements?
- Find some evidence from the literature at the end of this chapter to support your opinions.

Diagnosing readiness to learn

[Readiness] is a state of mind which reflects the outcome of quite a lot of psychological activity. For example, one difference between a child who refuses to go to school, another who dithers on the doorstep and a third who leaps enthusiastically onto the school bus is clear-cut: they differ in their readiness. (Rollnick et al., 2002, p. 18)

Anyone with an interest in health psychology and behavioural change (DiClemente & Prochaska, 1998) will be quick to draw parallels between the readiness of clients and patients to attempt changes in their health-related behaviour, and the readiness of learners to attempt new learning. Two concepts that stand out in explanations of patients' readiness to change are importance (how much importance does the individual attach to making the change?) and self-efficacy (how strong is the individual's belief that he or she is capable of making the change?). These concepts apply equally well to learners approaching a new learning experience.

One advantage of learning agreements is that the negotiation process is enormously helpful in enabling practice-based educators to acquire enough information to decide how receptive a learner is to embarking on a learning experience and how willing and able he or she feels to participate in the process. How ready learners are to progress along the practice learning continuum (Figure 6.4) can also be revealed by, for example, working alongside you with patients, through your observation, questioning and informal discussions. All these ongoing activities provide clues about learning readiness and enable you, as educator, to respond appropriately (Scully & Shepard, 1983).

> As a result of our informal discussion I realised that I was asking too much of my learner who needed help to prioritise their caseload . . . if I had not made time for them to discuss their concerns they would have lost confidence. (a practice-based educator)

Frameworks for diagnosing learning readiness

A search of the Internet reveals any number of self-assessment inventories that can be used to assess one's readiness for different types of learning. Distance learning and e-learning are two examples. For our purposes, a simple framework of factors likely to influence learning readiness is shown in Box 6.4. As you will see, it provides some useful additional prompt questions upon which to base learning agreement negotiations.

If you have not done so already, now would be a good time to read Chapter 4, 'The practice-based learning environment: social context and relationships'.

Using demonstration to facilitate learning

Facilitating clinical skills acquisition in the practice setting is a key activity for practice-based educators. As skilled practitioners, you may be working with undergraduates or novices who are performing therapeutic techniques or psychomotor skills for the first time, or only after practising in a simulated environment, such as a clinical skills laboratory. Alternatively, you may be working with experienced practitioners who are developing their expertise

---

Box 6.4. Factors influencing learning readiness

Past experience
Has the learner had previous experiences in similar locations that mean learning will come more easily in the new setting?

Health status
Could illness or other physical or emotional impairments interfere with progress or the capacity to acquire new skills in the time available? How can these be accommodated?

Environmental effects
Does the learner perceive the environment to be welcoming and conducive to learning? Is accessing the practice location straightforward or problematic? How can difficulties be accommodated?

Anxiety level
Is the learner's anxiety level compatible with learning? A degree of anxiety is a stimulus to learning. Too low a level (for example due to lack of interest and motivation) or too high a level (for example caused by fear of failure or marked cultural differences) will inhibit ready involvement in the learning process.

Locus of control
How self-directed is the learner? Is he or she keen to grasp control of the learning process (intrinsically motivated)? Is he or she relying on the practice-based educator to provide the stimulus to engage (extrinsically motivated)?

Knowledge base
How much does the learner already know about the practice area? How proficient is the learner in relevant skills?

Learning style
Does the ethos of the practice setting fit comfortably with the learner's preferred style of learning? Does he or she need help to attempt different approaches?

---

to a more advanced level. In either case, by structuring learning through demonstration the practice-based educator has four main goals (Cox, 1988). These are to demonstrate:

- communication skills: building the patient's confidence and trust, eliciting her/his expectations, understanding and responses;
- perceptual skills: active exploration and search for information through seeing, hearing, smelling and touching available evidence of dysfunction or disease;
- reasoning skills: interpreting findings, recognising patterns, generating and testing likely explanations and hypotheses;
- manual/procedural skills: applying relevant examination and/or therapeutic techniques.

During the demonstration, the learner has three main goals (Cox, 1988). These are to:

- observe the patient, the educator, and the clinical setting;
- participate actively by asking and responding to questions;
- learn the technique/procedure.

Using demonstration to develop reflective skills

Schon (1987) describes three ways to use demonstration as a method of reflection-in-action: they are 'follow me', 'joint experimentation', and 'hall of mirrors'. These three approaches have proved valuable in developing reflective skills for both practice-based educators and learners in healthcare settings (Alsop & Ryan, 1996).

Follow me is useful in the early stage of the practice development continuum. It can be linked to structured observation (see below). The key stages of 'follow me' are as follows:

1. The practice educator demonstrates a whole piece of practice, for example an aspect of a patient assessment, while the learner watches and makes notes of key points observed during the interaction.
2. The educator repeats the demonstration but stops at times to emphasise specific points of importance for the learner, for example to explain the reasoning behind particular probing questions directed at the patient. During this phase, the learner is encouraged to ask questions based on her/his initial observations.
3. The educator repeats the whole piece of practice without interruption, enabling the learner to observe again with more informed insight.

Joint experimentation is useful for practitioners seeking to develop more advanced skills and knowledge.

1. Initially the practice educator takes the lead.
2. At some part in the process, the educator stops and seeks the learner's opinion on how to proceed.
3. The educator proceeds with the task following the learner's suggestions and stops at a key point to discuss the outcomes of the learner's suggestions and to evaluate their effectiveness.
4. Learning is progressed by examining clinical reasoning in a series of supported steps.

In the **hall of mirrors**, either the learner or the educator performs the skill. At a key point, the procedure stops and a reflective discussion ensues. Ideally, this includes the patient (or a peer acting as a model). The learner is encouraged to think about feelings and to identify any challenges experienced when carrying out the skill, and receives feedback from both educator and patient.

Follow me, **joint experimentation** and **hall of mirrors** are good examples of a concept introduced earlier in the chapter. What is it?
Check back to p. 94 if you can't make the link.

EXPLORATORY REFLECTION 6.7

Think of a clinical skill or technique you might wish to demonstrate. Make a list of as many points as possible you might want to get over to learners during your demonstration. Categorise the points under the following headings:

- Communication skills
- Perceptual skills
- Reasoning skills
- Manual skills.

What questions do you think learners are most likely to ask during the demonstration?

Providing opportunities for structured observation

The range of what we think and do is limited by what we fail to notice. And because we fail to notice that we fail to notice, there is little we can do to change; until we notice how failing to notice shapes our thoughts and deeds. (Laing, 2005)

Boud and Walker (1998) emphasise the importance of learners actively noticing in order to learn from the activities and people they engage with in the practice setting. However, clinical practice is a complex and stressful environment for learners. The assault on their senses can be considerable, and this may be exacerbated by anxiety about not knowing enough, fear of failure and information overload. Consequently, recall of previously well-learnt information may be blocked, impairing accurate analysis of what they are observing, and hence their ability to formulate useful and relevant questions (Roskell & Cross, 1998). Providing a structure (or advance organiser) for their observations can help to reduce anxiety and facilitate learners' active engagement in observation and demonstration sessions such as those described above.

Stengelhofen (1993) suggests providing a structure that:

- identifies clear aims for the observation in advance of the demonstration;
- provides a set of prompt questions that form a focus for observation;

- allows time for discussion and evaluation following the demonstration;
- encourages learners to write up and reflect on their observations.

Some prompt questions you might consider are:

- 'What evidence was there that the practitioner was listening actively to the patient?'
- 'How and why was questioning adapted during the patient interaction?'
- 'Which cues did the practitioner follow up and why?'
- 'What non-verbal communication did you observe during the interaction, and what effect did it have?'
- 'Did any aspects of the physical environment influence the interaction and how?'
- 'What key information was obtained after five minutes, after 15 minutes etc.?'

A structured framework provides a focus, enabling learners to adopt an active, rather than passive, role. Experienced educators have found structured observation particularly valuable as a means of facilitating learning in community practice settings, where the nature of the setting may prevent learners from getting as much hands-on experience as in other situations.

EXPLORATORY REFLECTION 6.8

Look back to the demonstration you planned in Exploratory Reflection 6.7.

- Identify the aims of the demonstration.
- Using the list of points you wish to get over as a basis, prepare some prompt questions for learners to consider as they observe the demonstration.

Make a list of some other situations in which learners might adopt the role of active observer, and for which you could help them devise their own advance organiser, for example during a case conference to enhance an understanding of the roles of interprofessional team members.

Questioning and discussion

I shall never know if my students have really learned something until they are made to articulate and defend their position, through question and discussion for example. I must ask 'what if' questions such as, 'What if this was an elderly man instead of a young woman?' (Wooliscroft, 2004, p. 31)

It will be clear by now that asking questions in one form or another is fundamental to the learning and facilitation process. Here we consider some ways to make the most effective use of questioning, both to facilitate learners and to help you as the practice educator gain information about their progress, learning needs and readiness to learn. (We consider this type of activity as a means of formative assessment in Chapter 7.)

Different types of questions

'Convergent' questions are those with one best or correct answer. Questions that have a number of possible correct answers are 'divergent'. Watts (1990) classifies these further into:

Convergent questions that ask the learner to: .

- recall specific facts, procedures or theories etc.;
- construct an answer by using information from memory or gained from some other resource.

Divergent questions that ask the learner to:

- originate ideas and suggest alternative explanations or approaches;
- express opinions and reactions about issues, outcomes or events.

EXPLORATORY REFLECTION 6.9

Listed in Box 6.5 are some questions that ask learners to recall information, construct an answer, originate ideas or express opinions. Also in the box is the hierarchy of cognitive learning outcomes described above in Box 6.1.

By posing questions that reflect different levels in the cognitive hierarchy, the practice-based educator can discover what stage learners have reached in their learning and make decisions about their readiness to move on, their need for revision or consolidation.

- What levels in the cognitive hierarchy do you think the questions listed reflect? Match the level to the question by placing the appropriate letter (a–f) in the box beside each question. (See footnote for the solution.)[1]
- Now construct some more specific questions based on your own area of expertise that reflect different levels in the cognitive hierarchy.
- To what levels in the hierarchy does this Exploratory Reflection relate, do you think?

---

[1] 1 = a, 2 = d, 3 = e, 4 = b, 5 = f, 6 = c, 7 = a, 8 = f, 9 = b, 10 = e, 11 = f, 12 = c, 13 = e, 14 = d.

Box 6.5. Different levels of questioning to facilitate learning

Match the questions 1–14 to the cognitive skill levels by writing the appropriate letter a–f in the box beside each question.

Cognitive skill level

1. What is the normal value of . . . ?   □

2. What conclusions can you draw . . . ?   □

3. How would you modify this in order to . . . ?   □

4. Can you explain what's happening . . . ?   □

5. Should you accept the explanation that . . . ?   □

6. What questions would you ask in an interview with . . . ?   □

7. What comes next . . . ?   □

8. How effective is that . . . ?   □

9. Why does . . . usually produce . . . ?   □

10. How could you use . . . to . . . ?   □

11. How do you feel about . . . ?   □

12. What approach would you use to . . . ?   □

13. Using what you've learned, how would you set about . . . ?   □

14. Is this the same as . . . ?   □

Cognitive skill levels

a. KNOWLEDGE

b. UNDERSTANDING

c. APPLICATION

d. ANALYSIS

e. SYNTHESIS

f. EVALUATION

The importance of discussion

Of course, questions (the educator's or the learner's) can (and probably should) lead to conversation or discussion. Soden (1993, p. 18) points out that the best way of 'remedying thinking errors is to discuss them with someone else'. Often these learning conversations occur informally, during break times or while travelling between locations. It is important to acknowledge the challenge such conversations can pose for the practice-based educator, as well as their benefits for learners.

> Where the conversation may go is unpredictable. Such discussions often lead to areas where my own understanding is less than complete ... I have then to be willing to recognize the limits of my understanding and model the commitment to learn. (Wooliscroft, 2004, p. 31)

EXPLORATORY REFLECTION 6.10

- How aware are you of providing a role model of the commitment to learn as well as a role model of good clinical practice?
- In what ways do you demonstrate your commitment to learn?

Giving feedback

Moving forward in any learning situation is difficult without a clear idea of how well you are doing (Forster & Hounsell, 1995). The art of giving feedback lies in providing learners with accurate and useful information about good and poor aspects of their performance or behaviour, while at the same time motivating them to continue learning, improve their performance and seek further feedback.

> Feedback from a caring teacher is the most valuable ... resource, unfortunately it is one of the most poorly and infrequently used. (Wood, 2000, p. 19)

In health care there is a tendency always to expect very high standards. Therefore, if learners are doing well it is only to be expected and praise is given sparingly (ANZCA, 2002). This has unfortunate consequences for practitioners who:

- learn to focus on negative aspects rather than their performance as a whole;
- come to feel that positive feedback is inappropriate, hence tend to withhold praise in their dealings with learners and peers;
- find they have difficulty recognising and articulating their own personal strengths and exceptional qualities.

Undue concentration on negative aspects, unbalanced by any identification of positive aspects, can lead to anxiety, fear, lack of openness, loss of confidence, reduced learning, avoidance of issues and reluctance to seek further feedback (ANZCA, 2002). Provision of balanced feedback should be an ongoing process, rather than a freestanding item. It should be an integral and empowering part of the whole learning experience, with all participants engaged actively in its delivery.

EXPLORATORY REFLECTION 6.11   Try to recall a feedback experience that was particularly powerful for you as a learner in the practice setting.

- Describe the incident.
- Identify your own thoughts and feelings related to the feedback.
- How was the feedback delivered?
- Consider the language of the feedback. How did this impact on you as a learner?
- Analyse the incident and consider why it was so critical to your learning.
- Identify elements of good practice and areas for development related to the delivery and content of the feedback.
- How does your own approach to giving feedback to learners match up to your ideal?

Taras (2002) suggests that learners should be encouraged to self-assess before receiving feedback from their educator. This addition to the feedback cycle not only encourages learners to be more self-aware and self-critical but also gives educators insight into how learners feel about their progress. In Box 6.6, we have provided a checklist for giving effective feedback, and we return to the topic in Chapter 7, where we highlight its importance in both formative and summative assessment.

TOOLKIT SECTION TWO: FOSTERING COLLABORATION

Peer-assisted learning

Peer learning, or peer-assisted learning (PAL), refers to situations in which learners formally support each other in educational settings (Ashwin, 2002; Ladyshewsky, 2000). It is particularly relevant for initial healthcare programmes, since a rising demand for practice placements makes the traditional 1:1 model of practice-based education increasingly impracticable. Alternative practice-placement models involving two or more learners allocated to one practice-based educator make learners' appreciation of the need to support each other an important priority. This support may take a variety of forms along the cooperation–collaboration continuum described in Chapter 5 (p. 78). For example, learners might cooperate with each other by simply contributing discrete elements to a predefined group task. Alternatively, they

---

Box 6.6. Providing feedback for learners: a self-evaluation checklist

As a practice-based educator do I . . .

☐ establish a supportive environment encouraging learners to request feedback?

☐ agree when and how learners will be provided with feedback?

☐ begin by inviting the learner's self-assessment?

☐ as far as possible help learners make their own discoveries related to their practice?

☐ link my feedback to the negotiated learning outcomes whenever possible?

☐ always begin my feedback with positive observations?

☐ avoid following my positive observations with 'but' and a negative observation?

☐ focus on learners' behaviours and performances rather than making personal judgements about them?

☐ try to be as specific as possible, referring the learner to events I have observed when possible?

☐ give learners a language with which to reflect on their performance?

☐ attend to both what I say and how I say it?

☐ invite the learner to comment on the feedback?

☐ help learners turn negative feedback into constructive challenges?

☐ provide follow-up feedback when appropriate?

---

might collaborate in identifying practice-related problems and negotiating the means and processes for resolving them as a team (Figure 6.8).

EXPLORATORY REFLECTION 6.12   What do you see as the main effects of encouraging PAL? Discuss your views with a group of colleagues and learners.

Effects of PAL

The effects of any educational approach can be direct or indirect. Direct effects come from the content and skills involved in the learning activities. These are known as instructional effects. Indirect effects come from the environment created by the approach. These are known as 'nurturant effects'. Figure 6.9 shows some instructional and nurturant effects associated with PAL.

Cooperation

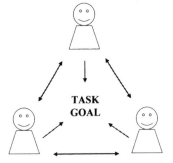

Discrete Contributions

TASK GOAL

Collaboration

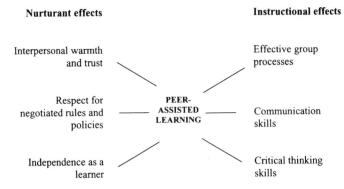

Figure 6.8. Peer cooperation and collaboration.

Nurturant effects   **Instructional effects**

Interpersonal warmth   Effective group
and trust   processes

Respect for   **PEER-**
negotiated rules and   **ASSISTED**   Communication
policies   **LEARNING**   skills

Independence as a   Critical thinking
learner   skills

Figure 6.9. Some effects of peer-assisted learning.

EXPLORATORY REFLECTION 6.13 In Table 6.1, we have listed some PAL activities alongside some advantages and comments from learners. Strategies for maximising the advantages are also listed. Discuss Table 6.1 with a group of colleagues and learners.

- Where do you think the activities sit along the cooperation–collaboration continuum?
- What nurturant and instructional effects do you think could emerge from the activities?
- Can you add to the list of suggestions for maximising the advantages of the PAL activities listed?

Instructional and nurturant effects are not necessarily positive. Therefore, when planning learning activities, it is important to ask ourselves whether the likely instructional and/or nurturant effects are desirable or undesirable.

> For example, high competition towards a goal may directly spur achievement, but the effects of living in a competitive atmosphere may alienate people from each other. (Joyce *et al.*, 1992, p. 16)

EXPLORATORY REFLECTION 6.14 Table 6.2 lists some disadvantages of PAL alongside comments from learners and educators. Can you add to the list of suggestions for minimising negative instructional and/or nurturant effects?

Now read Ladyshewsky (2000) Peer-assisted learning in clinical education: a review of terms and learning principles. *Journal of Physical Therapy Education*, 14(2), 15–22.

Interprofessional learning and team-skills development

A team is a set of interpersonal relationships structured to achieve particular goals, and in all areas of professional practice teams are considered 'not only positive, but inevitable' (Johnson & Johnson, 1991, p. 435). Also inevitable is the policy shift towards interprofessional as well as uniprofessional teams in health care.

> The emphasis on multi-professional teams and clinical networks as the means of delivering a clear service-driven agenda for change has major implications for education. Education programmes must respond more readily and flexibly, and necessary changes in educational processes, in both classroom and practice settings, must be sustained, embedded and capable of widespread replication. (DH, 2001)

Table 6.1. Advantages of peer learning in the practice setting

Activities and advantages	Learners' comments	Suggestions for maximising advantages
Peer support • increased professional socialisation • learners feel more relaxed and confident • knowledge, ideas and resources are shared	*'It's nice to be with someone who's in the same boat.'* *'It helps to bounce ideas off each other.'*	Establish some joint goals that learners work on together, for example a joint case presentation, with each learner taking responsibility for one aspect of the whole presentation. Encourage joint attendance at team meetings, ward rounds etc. with learners sharing responsibility for providing you with feedback.
Peer coaching and feedback • clinical reasoning is improved • anxiety and stress are reduced	*'If I've been observed by another student I'm working with on the placement, I feel quite happy asking them what they thought of it.'*	Provide opportunities for peer observation, using the ideas suggested earlier in this chapter on p. 111. Encourage learners to question and give each other feedback using the guidelines in Boxes 6.4 and 6.5.
Peer practice • newly acquired skills are practised more frequently • new knowledge is retained more easily because of frequent rehearsal	*'We had protected time to go off and practise together, which was really helpful.'*	Provide opportunities for learners to review knowledge and practise clinical skills together.
Peer reflection and evaluation • learners are stimulated to describe their experiential learning • tacit learning is made explicit	*'I think I probably reflected more when there were two of us. We'd talk about problems and issues and what we might do in the future.'*	Actively support learners' efforts to reflect on clinical cases and practice experiences together, share key incidents and describe learning that has emerged from problems they have faced. Encourage them to keep a record of their reflective conversations.

Table 6.2. Disadvantages of peer learning in the practice setting

Disadvantages	Learners' and educators' comments	Suggestions for maximising advantages
Managing individual differences may be difficult, for example in personality, ability, prior experience, culture, expectations etc.	*'You need to give that non-high-flyer personal time with you so that they can actually say, "I'm finding this difficult".'* (Educator)	• Allow time for individual feedback in private, when necessary. • Issues of different expectations may be raised during joint tutorials.
Competition between learners can lead to alienation.	*'I think if you are with another student who is competitive it might become an issue.'* (Learner)	• Identify some joint goals that learners can work towards together. • Ensure learners have some individual time with patients. • When working together, ensure learners alternate the roles of 'leader' and 'assistant'.
The overall caseload might be insufficient to satisfy the needs of several learners.	*'When it comes to caseload, we have to give junior staff priority over learners.'* (Educator)	• Involve other team members in planning learning experiences.
Space may be limited.		• Consider all possible learning experiences, for example visits to other disciplines, locations etc.
Learners may become isolated from the team.	*'We felt isolated from the staff because we couldn't all fit in the staffroom.'* (Learners)	• Encourage all team members to get to know learners and be involved with their learning experiences, where possible.

As the following comments demonstrate, campus-based interprofessional learning does not necessarily translate into interprofessional team working in the practice setting.

In college, you learn to become a specific professional, not a team member . . .
You learn from role models in the practice setting.
Learning about the roles of team members is more interesting and pertinent in the practice setting.
I've learnt from other people's experiences.

High-profile adverse events in health care have highlighted the need to dismantle barriers to interprofessional collaboration and team working, such as professional stereotyping and tribalism. The foundations of these barriers can be laid very early in a professional career (Hind *et al.*, 2003; Carpenter, 1995). Creating and utilising interprofessional learning opportunities to the full enables practice-based educators to negate such influences and foster a culture of collaboration across professions.

EXPLORATORY REFLECTION 6.15

What do you understand by the terms 'professional stereotyping' and 'tribalism'?

- Do you detect any evidence of stereotyping or tribalism in the network of colleagues that work together to provide quality health care in your particular practice context?
- To what extent does each member of the team understand and appreciate the specific ways in which the others contribute to patient care?
- What implicit messages about interprofessional team working do you think learners receive when they work in your practice context?

While exploring the extent of team-skills development in an initial healthcare education programme, Hilton and Morris (2001) noted that students attributed great importance to the skills of the practice-based educator in planning and offering interprofessional learning activities. Also, they felt 'held back' in their team-skills development when denied opportunities for independence and active collaboration.

EXPLORATORY REFLECTION 6.16

Hilton and Morris (2001) have developed a hierarchy of team-skills development (Table 6.3).

- Are elements of the team-skills development hierarchy represented in prescribed learning outcomes for learners on placement in your area (for example those laid down by the university or college)?
- Are they represented in learning agreements you have negotiated with learners?
- Do you think it would be useful to include them in future negotiations with learners?
- What specific opportunities exist for practice-based learners to gain interprofessional awareness and develop team skills in your practice context?

Opportunities for talking, observing and working alongside people with more or different expertise through case conferences, team meetings, ward rounds, discharge planning meetings, domiciliary visits and professional

Table 6.3. A hierarchy of team-skills development

Knowledge	Skills	Attitudes
Level One		
Demonstrate interprofessional awareness. Discuss the educational background and professional goals of various members of the healthcare team. Understand what other professionals know and do.	Demonstrate willingness and ability to: • communicate with other healthcare professionals; • teach professional skills to other healthcare professional students.	Appreciate the provision of health care as an interprofessional team function. Accept that opinions of colleagues are as valid as their own.
Level Two		
Identify areas of unique responsibility for each member of the team and areas of overlap.	Gather patient data and analyse it. Participate actively in cooperative goal structuring in relation to patient care. Collaborate and negotiate with colleagues as and when appropriate.	Value the opinions of colleagues. Be willing to give, receive and share information. Appreciate that complex patient problems demand an interprofessional approach.
Level Three		
	Work collaboratively to identify the total health needs of patients or client groups. Utilise a variety of cognitive and interpersonal skills to analyse and solve problems. Plan and initiate appropriate interventions as part of a team approach to healthcare provision. Generate evidence of critical reflection and evaluation of the team contribution to healthcare provision.	

conversations with colleagues and peers in other disciplines are some you may have identified.

Team models of practice education

Team models of practice education, in which the whole team (rather than only senior level experts) is encouraged to take some responsibility for a learner or group of learners in the practice setting, can help in team-skills development, and also provide an alternative way of accommodating multiple learners (Bennett, 2003; Baldry Currens & Bithell, 2000). Sharing responsibility for facilitating learners amongst all team members allows learners to experience different approaches to practice delivery and can have positive benefits for practitioners at all levels. Team skills are fostered as the educational skills of more junior staff are developed in a supportive way. If the prime educator is absent, other team members are available and personality conflicts between an educator and a learner can be more easily defused. However, care must be taken to ensure that there is a named lead educator and that communication channels are transparent and rigorous, ensuring learners feel adequately supported.

Clearly, collaboration between campus-based and practice-based educators in planning learner involvement in such activities is key to their successful implementation. In both settings, learners should be encouraged to reflect on their experiences of interprofessional learning and working and utilise them for role-development purposes.

At this point you may wish to read Hilton and Morris (2001) Student placement: is there evidence supporting team-skills development in clinical practice settings? *Journal of Interprofessional Care*, 15(2), 171–183.

Problem-based learning

Problem-based learning (PBL) could be thought of as the educator's 'Swiss army knife'. Potentially, it is one of the most multifunctional tools in the toolkit because, used appropriately, it can facilitate self-direction and peer-learning, team-working, critical-thinking and problem-solving skills, to name but a few.

PBL is different from presenting learners with problem-solving scenarios designed to test what they already know or have been taught. The focus of such scenarios is on demonstrating competence in a clearly defined area; there is no expectation that learners will explore much material beyond what is provided or readily available. PBL is designed to reveal to learners what they do not know but must find out in order to identify what the problem actually is, and go on to resolve it effectively. In other words, PBL does not test knowledge or skills, rather these are acquired and utilised simultaneously through the process of PBL.

> In problem-based learning environments [learners] act as professionals and confront problems as they occur – with fuzzy edges, insufficient information, and a need to determine the best solution possible by a given date. This is the manner in which engineers, doctors and . . . teachers, approach problem solving . . . unlike classrooms where teachers . . . guide students to neat solutions to contrived problems. (SCORE, 2004)

In the practice setting, the general aims of PBL are to (Sadlo, 1994):

- expand and deepen knowledge
- facilitate clinical-reasoning skills
- develop self-directed learning skills
- promote team learning skills.

PBL may be used in the practice setting to promote clinical reasoning by encouraging a small group or pair of learners to explore a real 'problem' from practice, for example a new referral to the department. It is particularly suitable for interprofessional learning in the practice environment, for example devising multidisciplinary and evidence-based care pathways. Such an approach enables learners to identify gaps in their understanding of a case and seek answers for themselves rather than rely solely on the educator's expertise. Presented with a case at the start of a placement, they work as a group to define the problem(s), gather information and postulate and test out hypotheses in order to reach a resolution by the end of the placement. Several issues may underpin the reasoning process, such as sociocultural context, epidemiology, pathogenesis, anatomy, psychology, legislation, departmental/ organisational constraints or imperatives etc. Individuals within the group will be responsible for exploring and feeding back on specific issues to help build the evidence base for an eventual resolution of the problem. At the end of the placement, the group may give a case presentation to the wider team, which should include a clear account of the evidence base underlying their analysis and ultimate resolution of the problem(s).

PBL and practice-based assessment

By collaborating to arrive at a successful resolution of a practice-based problem through PBL, learners also provide you, the educator, with evidence of their relative success in acquiring and applying relevant knowledge, skills and attitudes. As you monitor their progress at a distance, you will be gathering information that informs your formative feedback to learners, as well as your summative assessment decisions.

EXPLORATORY REFLECTION 6.17

- Have you used PBL with learners? If so, what are your feelings about it?
- Look back in the chapter to Boxes 6.1 and 6.2, and Table 6.3. With a group of colleagues and learners, discuss the relative value of PBL in fostering the knowledge, skills and attitudes listed, compared with other approaches to learning in the practice setting.
- If you have not used PBL before, would you consider using it? Discuss the reasons for your answer.

At this point, you might find it interesting to read the following critique of problem-based learning:

Morris (2003) How strong is the case for the adoption of problem-based learning in physiotherapy education in the United Kingdom? *Medical Teacher*, 25(1), 24–31.

TOOLKIT SECTION THREE: PROMOTING EMPOWERMENT

Challenge and support

As Figure 6.4 illustrates, promoting a real sense of empowerment in learners becomes increasingly important as they advance through a learning experience. By this we mean they demonstrate self-confidence and control over the practice environment, being able to place greater reliance on their own experience and judgement as reference points for action and decision-making. Eraut (2004), a prolific author on how professionals learn at work, describes four key types of professional activity which, when combined into an integrated performance, highlight the formidable challenge facing learners in the practice environment. The activities are:

- assessing clients and situations and continuing to monitor their condition;
- deciding what, if any, action to take, both immediately and over a longer period (either alone or as a leader or team member);
- pursuing an agreed course of action, modifying consulting and reassessing as and when necessary;
- managing oneself, one's job and one's continuing learning in a context of constrained time and resources, conflicting priorities and complex inter and intraprofessional relationships.

EXPLORATORY REFLECTION 6.18

- Compare Eraut's key professional activities with the skills and abilities you identified in Exploratory Reflection 6.2 and in the component activities of professional practice in Figure 6.1.
- How do your ideas fit into Eraut's conceptualisation?

Eraut's description of professional activity gives a good sense of the pace and pressure of the practice-based environment. It is a truism in education that sailing in calm waters doesn't teach (Valkeavaara, 1999). Therefore, exposing learners progressively to appropriate amounts of turbulence, or challenge, is fundamental to their empowerment as learners and practitioners.

EXPLORATORY REFLECTION 6.19

In Chapter 4 (p. 58), we considered the importance of trust in the learning environment. Look at that section again. In particular, consider your responses to Exploratory Reflection 4.4.

From your reading, you may have been struck by:

- the dynamic relationship between challenge and support in your role as a practice-based educator;
- the importance of effective use of challenge to move learners forward.

In Figure 6.10, we have adapted Daloz's (1999) model of the dynamic relationship between challenge and support.

- 'Low challenge, low support' provides no impetus for development. Nothing much happens and things stay as they are.
- 'Low challenge, high support' provides a low-risk, confirmatory environment in which learners can feel good about themselves. But while they are confirmed in their own actions, they may not be encouraged to acknowledge the legitimacy of other perspectives and viewpoints.
- 'High challenge, low support' causes disempowerment and drives learners into retreat. They may become trapped in a vicious circle of poor performance, negative feedback and negative feelings about their own abilities (Tang, 2003).
- 'High challenge, high support' in an appropriate mix are conducive to empowerment and professional growth. Learners feel empowered to step into the unknown and take appropriate risks with their learning.

EXPLORATORY REFLECTION 6.20

- Think about your own experiences as a learner. Can you map them onto the four quadrants in Figure 6.10?

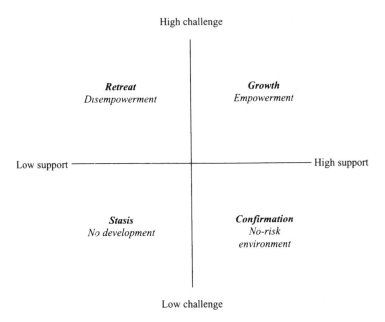

Figure 6.10. Relationship between challenge and support (adapted from Daloz, 1999).

- How do you think learners would map their experiences of working with you?

Cognitive dissonance

While support could be thought of as helping learners to close gaps by, for example, providing structure, acting as an advocate, sharing personal experiences etc., challenge is about deliberately opening up gaps that learners are then driven to close. In social science terms, this is known as creating 'cognitive dissonance'. According to the originator of the term (Festinger, 1957), learning occurs in response to learners' intrinsic need to act to dispel dissonance when it occurs. (You might want to link this bit of theory to those in Chapter 5.)

Creating cognitive dissonance

As a practice-based educator you can create cognitive dissonance in a number of ways.

- Set ambiguous tasks that cause uncertainty and confusion in learners, because you hold a perspective they have yet to develop.

- Combine ambiguous tasks with critical discussion that challenges learners to achieve deep learning through metacognition. (Remember this from Chapter 5? Look back to p. 83 if you can't make the link.)
- 'Heat up dichotomies' (Daloz, 1999) by challenging learners to recognise and value the legitimacy of different perspectives, to consider each viewpoint or approach and give each its due before taking a stand.

It's a long way from 'Our ways are right, theirs are wrong' to 'Our ways are sensible, theirs are quaint', to 'Our ways make sense to us, theirs to them; we differ because our worlds differ'. (Daloz, 1999, pp. 220–221)

- Construct hypotheses that challenge assumptions – 'What if . . .?' 'Suppose that . . .' 'Let's assume . . .'
- Set high standards. Expressing high, but realistic expectations for learners helps them raise their own expectations of themselves. 'I am here . . . I could be there . . .'

EXPLORATORY REFLECTION 6.21

These ideas for providing learners with appropriate challenges may well have caused you to ask some questions related to earlier sections of this chapter, for example:

- Are your own and their high expectations for learners reflected in the learning outcomes you negotiate with them?
- Are your questions to learners sufficiently challenging to reflect your own and their expectations, and the stage of the learning experience?
- Are you optimising the potential of problem-based learning and team learning to heat up dichotomies, develop new perspectives and enhance metacognitive skills?

Look again at Boxes 6.1–6.3 and 6.5 to remind yourself what you and learners are aiming for.

Learning relationships

Including learning relationships in the toolkit highlights the fact that where you choose to stand in relation to learners can act as a stimulus or a brake on learning. Figure 6.3 suggests that learning relationships evolve over time. Thus, a didactic relationship, in which you have greatest influence on developing the practice-based learning agenda and control over clinical decision-making, gradually evolves into a position of shared responsibility for decision-making and performance. Finally, you create distance in the relationship by adopting a more consultative (as opposed to collaborative) position. Here, you respond when requested by more empowered learners, to their narrowly defined, carefully formulated questions about patients for whom they take responsibility. (Depending on the context and level of the learner, this responsibility might be notional.) However, it is important to think of educational relationships on a continuum with movement possible in either direction.

> Overemphasis on one type of relationship at any given stage . . . can be inappropriate. For example, if the ability to solve problems is most important, then exclusive use of didactic relationships may encourage passivity and dependency, and not help [learners] acquire desired skills and independence. The reverse is also possible: an [educator] may remain in excessively consultative mode when the learner needs information or a demonstration . . . or supervision to acquire a new skill. (Magill *et al.*, 1986, p. 151)

Difficulties with learning relationships

Learning relationships reflect varying levels of power and responsibility. Empowered learners are able to exercise a measure of appropriate control over learning relationships based on their own analysis and assessment of their learning needs and abilities at any particular time. However, relationships with individual learners can pose problems.

EXPLORATORY REFLECTION 6.22

Discuss your experience of learning relationships with a group of colleagues.

- Have you ever been faced with a learner attempting to establish a consultative relationship too early, before you have sufficient confidence in her/his basic skills?
- Conversely, have you experienced learners reluctant to engage in a consultative relationship when this is a reasonable expectation?
- Do you feel sufficiently flexible in your use of learning relationships to be able to respond to varying learner needs?

In the 'troubleshooting' section of the toolkit (see below), we consider some factors that interfere with productive learning relationships and how you might deal with them.

Portfolio development

A portfolio is:

> . . . a private collection of evidence, which demonstrates the continuing acquisition of skills, knowledge, attitudes, understanding and achievement. It is both retrospective and prospective, as well as reflecting the current stage of development of the individual. (Brown, 1992, p. 2)

A personal portfolio is the larger resource from which specific pieces of evidence may be selected to make up a smaller profile for a particular purpose or audience, for example a work-based appraisal or a job interview. There are a number of reasons why portfolio development is an important tool in your task of empowering learners.

Portfolios and lifelong learning

In Chapter 5, we included in the characteristics of self-directed learners the ability to 'cope with ambiguity, uncertainty and change,' (p. 77). Certainly, high levels of adaptability, flexibility and responsiveness to change are essential for survival and career satisfaction in the healthcare professions. The term used to describe this combination is lifelong learning. Lifelong learners are described (ENB, 1995; Hull & Redfern, 1996) as being:

- innovative in their practice;
- flexible to changing demand;
- resourceful in their methods of working;
- able to work as change agents;
- able to share good practice and knowledge;
- adaptable to changing healthcare needs;
- challenging and creative in their practice;
- self-reliant in their way of working;
- responsible and accountable for their work.

The pace and pressure of healthcare practice mean the responsibility for developing these characteristics lies with individuals through their own self-direction as learners. Portfolios serve as the repository of evidence of their achievement.

Portfolios and appraisal

Work-based appraisal in the health professions is a formal process designed to support high-quality patient care and improve clinical standards (Chambers et al., 2003). It should be:

> ... a positive process to give someone feedback on their performance, to chart their continuing progress and to identify development needs ... it is a forward-looking process ... to help consolidate and improve on good performance aiming towards excellence. (Chambers et al., 2003, p. 3)

Making clear your expectation of high-quality evidence of learning, for example through learning agreements, will help empower learners to engage effectively with appraisal. As a result, they will be able to negotiate meaningful professional development plans that benefit them as individuals, as well as the wider service.

EXPLORATORY REFLECTION 6.23

- Spend some time looking through your own personal portfolio. What evidence is there that you possess the characteristics of an effective lifelong learner?
- How might the portfolio sheets provided in this book contribute to your evidence?
- How do you make it clear to learners that you value the process of portfolio development?

TOOLKIT SECTION FOUR: TROUBLESHOOTING

Bearing in mind Brookfield's (1986, p. 294) description of learning interactions as 'psychosocial dramas' (see Chapter 4), it is hardly surprising that, despite our best endeavours, things do not always progess smoothly. You may recall that in Chapter 5 we pointed out that understanding learning theory helps educators to adopt an objective stance when things go wrong. Being able to draw on learning theory:

> . . . helps practitioners realise that what might seem like signs of their own personal inadequacies as educators can often be interpreted as inevitable consequences of a host of other factors. (Chapter 5, p. 70)

In this section of the toolkit we illustrate the usefulness of theoretical frameworks in solving problems associated with learning, facilitation and learning relationships, with the help of the six vignettes shown in Box 6.7.

First of all, we use Vignettes 1–4 to illustrate some common problems that occur in the interaction between practice-based educators and learners. We analyse these problems in terms of what they tell us about

- learner alienation in the practice-based learning environment;
- match and mismatch between learner stage of development and educator approach;
- fear and failure in the practice-based learning enviroment.

Secondly, we consider how these four problems might be alleviated through enhanced communication and dialogue. Finally, we use Vignettes 4 and 5 to explore the idea of the 'blocked learning cycle' and suggest some ideas for helping learners who have become blocked at different stages.

Box 6.7. Problems with practice-based learning interactions

Vignette 1

An undergraduate from overseas appears over-confident and rarely asks for help or advice. The practice-based educator has little confidence in this learner's basic skills and suspects he is 'winging it' a lot of the time.

Vignette 2

Four graduate learners on an accelerated masters degree qualifying programme are together on a 4:1 practice placement. Their practice-based educator has experience of working in 1:1 relationships with traditional undergraduates. She finds working with the graduate learners very stressful. They appear to be uncooperative and not prepared to get on with the tasks assigned to them. They distract the educator with a lot of questions and challenge some of the information they are given. The educator resents being put under this sort of pressure. The learners find her unfriendly and don't feel they have any choices about their learning experiences. Their opinions are not valued and they are not learning anything.

Vignette 3

A group of junior practitioners on rotation in the same specialty are encouraged by the senior practitioner to plan a programme of in-service education to facilitate their development during the rotation. They are expected to draw up a list of skills-development needs and some ideas about how they can work together to address these. The novices are not particularly enthusiastic about this. They say they have little time to get together to discuss things, and anyway they are too inexperienced in the specialty to decide what they really need to work on. They think the senior is in a better position to decide on content and run the sessions. They feel they are not getting the support they need.

Vignette 4

An undergraduate learner and practice-based educator are discussing the results of the learner's end-of-placement assessment. Although the overall grade is not a fail, the learner is upset by the assessment; his expectations were much higher. He says that insufficient feedback from the practice-based educator was the reason for his poor performance. He could not be expected to know where he was going wrong. Later, the educator's colleagues tell her that, in their opinion, she should have failed the learner because his performance had been consistently poor.

Vignette 5

A mature learner on a placement in a neurological intensive care setting seems detached and uninterested. She is slow to take advantage of opportunities to observe procedures in the operating theatre or to spend time with qualified staff assisting in the management of patients in the unit. In discussion with the learner, the practice educator discovers that she is the mother of a young adult of a similar age to the patients in the unit. The association between the patients and her own son make it very difficult for her to remain detached and cope with the emotional stress of immersing herself fully in this particular learning opportunity.

Vignette 6

Patients and staff on an elderly care rehabilitation ward all agree one learner has 'the gift of the gab'. He spends a lot of time chatting and seems interested in people's lives and concerns. In case conferences he is confident in discussing socioeconomic and political issues. As far as the practice educator is concerned, the learner produces little in the way of objective assessment or worthwhile rehabilitation outcomes that will optimise his patients' return to functional independence. After sharing her concerns with the learner's visiting academic tutor, she discovers that he has a history of failing to commit time and energy to practising new skills or translating theory into practice.

Learner alienation in the practice-based learning environment

The experience of alienation can be described as one in which:

> [Learners feel] unable to engage or contribute in ways which are meaningful and productive for the realisation of their own potential and learning requirements. (Mann, 2005, p. 43)

In Vignettes 1–4 one common factor constraining learners' ability to engage or contribute is the assumptions that they and their educators make about each other and/or the learning environment.

EXPLORATORY REFLECTION 6.24 Before reading on, decide what you consider to be the underlying assumption(s) being made by the participants in each of Vignettes 1–4.

In Vignette 1 one possibility is the learner's assumption that being a 'good learner' means being seen to be independent and always knowing what to do. Since he associates appearing uncertain and asking for help with poor performance, he is alienated from the possibility of acting positively to resolve difficulties he faces in his learning. Of course, another possibility is that he has an inflated notion of his own abilities (he doesn't know what he doesn't know). As a result, he is attempting to establish a consultative learning relationship before he is really ready to do so.

In Vignette 2 both parties seem to be making assumptions about the learning relationship but are unaware of each other's viewpoints. The learners seem to be seeking collaboration or shared responsibility with the educator. The educator is adopting a didactic approach. This lack of mutual awareness constrains their capacity to interact with each other and limits the extent of learners' participation.

Vignettes 3 and 4 both suggest assumptions about role and responsibility. Teaching and assessment are assumed by the learners to be the practice-based educator's responsibility, whereas, especially in Vignette 3, the educator has assumed learners' ability to take responsibility for themselves.

Match and mismatch between learner development and educator approach

In Chapter 5, we introduced the concept of learner development and discussed learners' readiness to move towards greater levels of self-direction. As a practice-based educator, you may find your instinctive tendency is to be more or less directive in your approach to learners. You might think of this as a continuum from a strict authoritarian approach to one of maximal delegation of responsibility to learners. However, a flexible approach is necessary if learners are to be empowered to develop. Thus, you might choose to match your approach to learners' stage of development or deliberately create a mismatch. Problems can arise when the mismatch is unplanned or inappropriate.

> To stimulate development we *deliberately* mismatch the [learner] and the environment so that the [learner] cannot easily maintain the familiar patterns, but must move on towards greater complexity. (But not too much so, for we seek an optimal mismatch where the learner's conceptual systems are challenged but not overwhelmed.) (Joyce *et al.*, 1992, p. 394, original emphasis)

EXPLORATORY REFLECTION 6.25

How aware are you of adapting your approach in order to:

- match learners' existing level of self-direction?
- move them on to increase their self-direction?

Vignette 2 suggests what can happen when learners capable of taking control of their learning are paired with an overly directive educator. Adults reentering higher education after life experiences and responsibility can find directive approaches difficult to deal with. While some remain able to function well and retain overall control of their learning, others rebel against what they see as low-level demands and retreat into boredom (Grow, 1996).

In Vignette 3 the opposite has occurred. The learners resent the educator for delegating a responsibility they do not feel ready to accept.

> ... wanting the reassuring presence of an authority figure telling them what to do [will mean that they] are unlikely to respond to the delegating style of a nice humanistic facilitator, hands-off delegator, or critical theorist who demands they confront their own learning roles. (Grow, 1996)

EXPLORATORY REFLECTION 6.26

Look back to Perry's hierarchy of learner development in Chapter 5, p. 73.

- What stage do you think the learners in Vignettes 2 and 3 have reached?
- What stage do you think their practice-based educators are expecting?

Fear and failure

Fear and failure are both key concepts in Vignettes 1–4.

In Vignette 1 the learner's fear of failure is based on his assumption of what it means to be a 'good learner'. Fear of failure or 'loss of face' causes learners to focus excessively on themselves and have difficulty opening themselves up to new experiences and ideas. This stands in the way of their development (De Weerdt *et al.*, 2002).

Vignette 2 illustrates the fears educators can feel when required to adapt their existing, ingrained skills in order to take on new or unfamiliar approaches to learning facilitation. Attempting to use new approaches generates considerable discomfort and anxiety that interferes with the development of productive relationships with learners.

In Vignette 3 fear of failure is linked to attribution of expertise. In other words, the learners avoid responsibility for their own development by hiding behind the expertise of the practice-based educator. This hiding only serves to perpetuate their fear (De Weerdt *et al.*, 2002).

In Vignette 4 the practice-based educator's fear of failing the learner is the issue. We consider the problems associated with awarding a 'fail' grade in Chapter 7, p. 170. For now, it is worth noting that, to most practice-based educators, the idea of failing learners in the practice environment seems strangely at odds with the:

• humanistic principles associated with andragogy,
• 'duty of care' practitioners extend from patients to include learners with whom they work.

Therefore, it is not surprising that fear of learners' reactions is foremost in the range of adverse emotions associated with assigning a fail grade.

EXPLORATORY   With a group of colleagues, discuss the extent
REFLECTION 6.27   to which fear has been a part of your experiences
                       as an educator and/or as a learner.

• What were the causes of your fear?
• How did you deal with/overcome it?

Enhancing communication and dialogue

Good interpersonal communication is fundamental to effective learning.

> ... we each construct our own meaning for the communication we send and receive ... the meaning of our communication is the response we get. (Waters *et al.*, 2005)

The responses provoked by the communication in Vignettes 1–4 all inhibit effective learning because the participants' personal perceptions are hidden from one another. They are constrained by the perceptions of reality they have constructed in their own minds based on their unsubstantiated assumptions.

In Section 1 of the Toolkit we looked at how the process of learning-needs analysis helps learners and practice-based educators reveal their respective needs and expectations to each other.

EXPLORATORY REFLECTION 6.28

- Look at the questions listed in the first part of the negotiation cycle shown in Figure 6.6.
- In light of the problems revealed in the vignettes, are there any additional questions you think should be added to the list for learners and educators?
  (See below for our suggestions.)

The Johari Window

This method of enhancing interpersonal awareness and communication takes its name from its originators, Joseph and Harry Ingham (Beach, 1982). Used appropriately, it can help to preempt the types of problems exemplified in the vignettes. Cross (1996) describes how the Johari Window can be applied to learning-needs analysis in the practice setting. Although at first this process might appear time-consuming, it is analogous to the thoroughness required for an initial assessment of patients. Without a clear analysis of clinical problems and patient expectations, the effectiveness and efficiency of subsequent interventions and management could be compromised and valuable time wasted in the long run.

Using the Johari Window for practice-based learning-needs analysis

Stage 1: Learner and practice-based educator begin by making separate lists of their personal needs, abilities, expectations and ideas in relation to the learning experience. This may be done some time in advance of the experience, and in effect forms an agenda for their first meeting. The questions in Figure 6.6 provide a useful starting point for compiling the lists. However, it is important to remember that learning needs are not only confined to clinical knowledge and skills. They also encompass knowledge and skills related to being a competent learner. Hence, in your reflection above you may have identified the following as important additional questions:

Learner:

- In what ways do I think I can take control of my own learning during this experience?
- What are my expectations of the practice-based educator in helping me to take control?
- How do I think the educator expects me to behave as a learner?

Educator:

- In what ways do I expect the learner(s) to take control of their own learning during this experience?

- In what ways am I willing and able to help them to take control?
- How do I think the learner(s) expect me to behave as a facilitator of their learning?

Stage 2: When learner and educator meet, they compare their lists and together they allocate their respective ideas, needs and expectations to the relevant panes of the Johari Window, as shown in Figure 6.11. Pane A represents the shared perceptions of learner and educator. It indicates where they are on the same wavelength. Any or all items in this area may be prioritised as a focus for learning outcome statements.

Panes B and C indicate where the educator and learner differ in their perceptions. This may result from lack of knowledge or awareness, or a difference of opinion. Items in these areas may be the focus of negotiation or discussion between educator and learner until they reach agreement about how they can be addressed constructively. However, if they relate to mandatory institutional expectations, they may have to be accepted as non-negotiable or prescribed. Other items in these two panes might prove resistant

	Known to learner (Shared area)	Not known to learner (Negotiated/prescribed area)
Known to practice educator	*A* Needs, abilities, expectations and ideas that appear on **BOTH** learner's and educator's lists	Needs, abilities, expectations and ideas that appear ONLY on the **EDUCATOR'S** list *B*
Not known to practice educator	Needs, abilities, expectations and ideas that appear ONLY on the **LEARNER'S** list *C*	Needs, abilities, expectations and ideas revealed as a **CONSEQUENCE** of the learning experience *D*
	(Negotiated/prescribed area)	(Revealed area)

Figure 6.11. Using the Johari Window as a basis for learning-needs analysis.

to negotiation for a variety of reasons. Rather than waste time and undermine the learning relationship, an 'agreement to differ' might be appropriate, with an undertaking to revisit the issues at a later date.

Pane D remains empty until the end of the experience when the learner will have gained new insights into her/his needs and abilities as well as practice demands. This pane provides:

- a stimulus for reflection and learning transfer;
- the starting point for a new list of needs, expectations and ideas relating to the negotiation of a subsequent learning agreement.

Advantages of the Johari Window

- It provides a legitimate framework (or risk-free zone) for learners to express their feelings and concerns without fear of censure or misunderstanding. Through this process, the educators in Vignettes 1 and 3 could have acquired a clearer idea of their learners' stage of development and been able to adjust the balance of challenge and support accordingly.
- It provides a legitimate opportunity for educators to engage in appropriate self-disclosure in order to facilitate dialogue. For example, by revealing her lack of experience with alternative placement models, the educator in Vignette 2 could invite the learners' collaboration in making the new arrangements work and facilitating her own development as an educator.
- The Johari Window is one way to optimise the whole process of negotiation of learning agreements, particularly in planning for formative and summative assessment (Vignette 4).

EXPLORATORY REFLECTION 6.29

- With a group of colleagues and learners, discuss the potential value of the Johari Window in facilitating communication and dialogue in your area(s) of practice.
- Consider its use with both individuals and groups. For example, how could it be used to optimise implementation of alternative placement models and team working?

The blocked learning cycle

So far we have thought about what can go wrong when communication breaks down in learning interactions and what can happen when assumptions are made that are not necessarily shared by all participants. Now we look at these issues another way by asking the question 'What happens when learners get blocked in the learning cycle?' using Vignettes 5 and 6 in Box 6.7 as illustrative examples.

In Chapter 5, we described a four-stage experiential learning cycle based on Kolb (1984) and pointed out that simply having experience is not the same thing as learning from it. Therefore, movement through all four stages of the learning cycle is necessary for effective learning and development to occur.

EXPLORATORY REFLECTION 6.30   Look back to Chapter 5, p. 74 to remind yourself of the activities involved in each stage of the experiential learning cycle.

Why do learners get blocked in the learning cycle?

Figure 6.12 illustrates the behaviours associated with learners becoming blocked at each stage of the learning cycle. Some learners may get blocked

Blocked at experiencing

- withdrawn and distant
- cynical/negative about new ideas
- fearful of involvement
- lacking confidence
- ambivalent about specialty/career choice

Blocked at experimenting

- hyperactive
- disorganised
- needs to be needed
- 'too busy' for reflective discussion
- defensive about justifying reasons for action

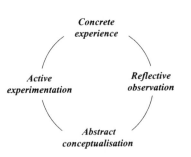

Blocked at reflection

- overanxious
- dependent
- constant discussion of feelings
- procrastination
- butterfly thinking

Blocked at conceptualising

- avoids feelings
- intellectualisation
- constant widening of issues
- uses theorising to block positive action

Figure 6.12. Behaviours associated with the blocked learning cycle (adapted from Morrison, 2001).

because of problems with a specific issue or clinical case; Vignette 5 is an example of this. Others may be blocked at a particular stage regardless of the issue (Vignette 6). Reasons for this can include time pressures, inappropriate balance of challenge and support from practice-based educators, stage of learning development, organisational or practice-based cultures that discourage some activities in the cycle, such as reflection or theorising, previous negative learning experiences or peer pressure. All these can be powerful inhibitors of movement through the cycle (Morrison, 2001).

Strategies to help learners unblock and move on

Box 6.8 lists some strategies you might find useful in helping learners to identify their problems with the learning cycle and become unblocked. As we have

---

Box 6.8. Strategies for dealing with blocks in the learning cycle
(adapted from Morrison, 2001)

When learners are blocked at experiencing:

- Explore how they feel about their progress and aspirations.
- Find out which areas of the learning experience are unsatisfying or disliked.
- Enquire sensitively whether there is anything else happening to distract them getting involved.
- Clarify your expectations about levels of skill and knowledge.
- Find out what they feel confident about.
- Discuss their developmental needs in detail.
- Make clear how you will provide constructive feedback and support.

When learners are blocked at experimenting:

- Find out how they are feeling about the pressures of the practice-based experience.
- Recognise their commitment and abilities.
- Help them analyse their time management.
- Ask them to summarise their activities and the rationale for their actions

When learners are blocked at reflecting:

- Explore how the task is similar to something else they have managed before, identifying positive and negative outcomes.
- Break the task down into manageable parts that match their own perceived level of competence.
- Prioritise what needs to be done and set time limits.
- Encourage them to specify the help they need from you or others.
- Provide an opportunity to practise beforehand.
- On completion of the task review what happened and help them analyse what went well and areas for development.

When learners are blocked at conceptualising:

- Remain focused on relevant issues and avoid being drawn into generalisations.
- Prioritise what needs to be achieved and set review dates.
- Give feedback if questions about feelings are answered with theoretical responses or generalisations.

already suggested, it is always a good idea to try to preempt problems through communication. Thus, using the learning cycle as a framework for discussing their learning history with learners at the start of a learning experience provides another means for practice-based educators and learners to build effective learning relationships and optimise learning opportunities.

EXPLORATORY REFLECTION 6.31

- At what stages in the experiential learning cycle are the learners in Vignettes 5 and 6 blocked?
- What strategies would you choose to unblock them?
- Have you ever found yourself blocked in the experiential learning cycle; if so, what behaviours did you demonstrate?
- What caused you to become blocked?
- Can you recognise any of the 'blocked behaviours' in learners or colleagues with whom you work?
- Discuss the idea of the 'blocked learning cycle' with colleagues. Are there other strategies for dealing with it that you could add to those in Box 6.8?

Summary

This chapter has explored a range of ideas and methods for facilitating learning in the practice setting. These are presented in the form of a 'flexible toolkit'. Important points to consider are:

- Effective facilitation draws on the principles of adult learning.
- Facilitation in the practice setting involves a developmental process of structuring learning, fostering collaboration and promoting independence in learners.
- Avoiding problems in learning, facilitation and learning relationships starts with sharing perceptions, assumptions and expectations.
- Together, practice-based learners and educators can explore and resolve problems associated with learning, facilitation and learning relationships by using appropriate models or frameworks such as the Johari Window and the experiential learning cycle.

Now complete the portfolio sheet for Chapter 6.

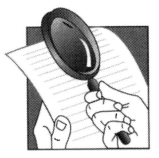

- Check how often you use aspects of learning theory to optimise your effectiveness as a practice-based educator.
- Consider what evidence you have of your ability to fulfil ACCREDITATION OUTCOME IV. Is it sufficient? If not, identify where the gaps lie and how they might be filled.
- Identify your continued development needs.

- Reassess your confidence in relation to Chapter 6's learning outcomes, including any personal learning outcomes you identified for yourself.
- Complete your action plan.

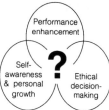

Finally, discuss the different ways in which Chapter 6 has helped you to think about your role as a practice-based educator. What reflective purposes has the chapter served for you?

Portfolio Sheet – Facilitating learning in the practice setting

Activities associated with effective facilitation of learning	Frequency of involvement			Development need?	
	Regularly	Occasionally	Never	YES	NO
Structuring learning					
Negotiating learning agreements	☐	☐	☐	☐	☐
Diagnosing readiness to learn	☐	☐	☐	☐	☐
Using different models of demonstration	☐	☐	☐	☐	☐
Providing opportunities for structured observation	☐	☐	☐	☐	☐
Strategic questioning and discussion	☐	☐	☐	☐	☐
Giving feedback	☐	☐	☐	☐	☐
Fostering collaboration					
Peer-assisted learning	☐	☐	☐	☐	☐
Interprofessional learning	☐	☐	☐	☐	☐
Team-skills development	☐	☐	☐	☐	☐
Problem-based learning	☐	☐	☐	☐	☐
Promoting independence					
Strategic use of challenge and support	☐	☐	☐	☐	☐
Introducing cognitive dissonance	☐	☐	☐	☐	☐
Using different types of learning relationships	☐	☐	☐	☐	☐
Encouraging portfolio development	☐	☐	☐	☐	☐
Troubleshooting					
Avoiding problems by sharing perceptions, assumptions and expectations	☐	☐	☐	☐	☐
Resolving problems using appropriate models	☐	☐	☐	☐	☐

Existing evidence for ACCREDITATION OUTCOME IV (give details)

Plan, implement and facilitate learning in the clinical setting

Sufficient evidence? YES ☐ NO ☐

Personal learning outcomes for Chapter 6

Confident   Not sure

ACTION PLAN

Chapter 6's Learning Outcomes

     I am confident I can do this   I am not sure I can do this

1. Discuss key principles underpinning facilitation of learning in the practice setting. ☐ ☐

2. Explain the significance of the relationship between practice-based educator and learner in the facilitation process. ☐ ☐

3. Select and justify the use of a range of methods to
   - plan and structure learning in the practice setting; ☐ ☐
   - foster collaboration between peers and teams; ☐ ☐
   - promote independence in practice-based learners. ☐ ☐

4. Employ appropriate strategies for avoiding and/or resolving problems associated with practice-based learning, facilitation and learning relationships. ☐ ☐

Bibliography

Allan J (2000) Does outcome-led design influence how students approach learning? *Capability: Journal of Autonomous Learning for Life and Work*, 4(2), 16–21.

Alsop A, Ryan S (1996) *Making the Most of Fieldwork Education: A Practical Approach*. London: Chapman & Hall, Chapter 15.

*Anderson G, Boud D, Sampson J (1996) *Learning Contracts: A Practical Guide*. London: Kogan Page.

Anderson JL (1988) The Supervisory Process in Speech-Language Pathology and Audiology. Boston: College Hill Press.

Ashwin P (2002) Implementing peer learning across organisations: the development of a model. *Mentoring & Tutoring*, 10(3), 221–231.

Australian and New Zealand College of Anaesthetists (ANZCA) (2002) Education & training modules: motivation <http://www.anzca.edu.au/emodules/2-motivation.htm> (accessed 20 July 2005).

Baldry Currens JA, Bithell CP (2000) Clinical education: listening to different perspectives. *Physiotherapy*, 86(12), 645–653.

Beach EK (1982) Johari's Window as a framework for needs assessment. *Journal of Continuing Education in Nursing*, 13(3), 28–32.

Bennett R (2003) Clinical education: perceived abilities/qualities of clinical educators and team supervision of students. *Physiotherapy*, 89(7), 432–440.

Bloom BS (1956) *Taxonomy of Educational Objectives, Handbook I: The Cognitive Domain*. New York: David McKay.

Boud D, Walker D (1998) Promoting reflection in professional courses: the challenge of context. *Studies in Higher Education*, 23(2), 191–206.

Brookfield S (1986) *Understanding and Facilitating Adult Learning*. Milton Keynes: Open University Press.

Brookfield S (1998) Critically reflective practice. *The Journal of Continuing Education in the Health Professions*, 18(4), 197–205.

Brown RA (1992) *Portfolio Development and Profiling for Nurses*. Lancaster: Quay Publishing.

Carpenter J (1995) Doctors and nurses: stereotypes and stereotype change in interprofessional education. *Journal of Interprofessional Care*, 9(2), 151–161.

Chambers R, Wakely G, Field S, Ellis S (2003) *Appraisal for the Apprehensive: A Guide for Doctors*. Abingdon: Radcliffe Medical Press.

Cox K (1988) How to teach at the bedside. In Cox KR, Ewan CE (eds), *The Medical Teacher*. London: Churchill Livingstone.

*Cross V (1996) Introducing learning contracts into physiotherapy clinical education. *Physiotherapy*, 82(1), 21–27.

**Daloz L (1999) *Mentor: Guiding the Journey of Adult Learners*. San Francisco: Jossey-Bass.

Dave   HR   (1970)   http://www.personal.psu.edu/staff/b/x/bxb11/Objectives/psychomotor.htm (accessed 19 February 2006).

Department of Health (2001) Common Learning: Information for stakeholders about inter professional education. <http://www.dh.gov.uk/PolicyAndGuidance/HumanResourcesAndTraining/LearningAndPersonalDevelopment/

PreRegistration/PreRegistrationArticle/fs/en?contentID=4052470&chk=i67cob>, accessed 22 July 2005.

De Weerdt S, Corthouts F, Martens H, Bouwen R (2002) Developing professional learning environments: model and application. *Studies in Continuing Education*, 24(1), 25–38.

DiClemente CC, Prochaska J (1998) Towards a comprehensive, transtheoretical model of change: stages of change and addictive behaviours. In Miller RW, Heather N (eds), *Treating Addictive Behaviours*. New York: Plenum.

English National Board for Nursing, Midwifery and Health Visiting (1995) Creating Lifelong Learners. Partnerships for Care: Guidelines for the implementation of the UKCC's Standards for Education and Partnership. London: ENB.

**Eraut M (2004) Informal learning in the workplace. *Studies in Continuing Education*, 26(2), 248–273.

Festinger L (1957) *A Theory of Cognitive Dissonance*. Stanford, CA: Stanford University Press.

Forster F, Hounsell D (1995) *Tutoring and Demonstrating: A Handbook*. University of Edinburgh: Centre for Teaching, Learning & Assessment.

Gilmartin J (2001) Teachers' understanding of facilitation styles with student nurses. *International Journal of Nursing Studies*, 38(4), 481–488.

Grant J (2002) Learning needs assessment: assessing the need. *British Medical Journal*, 324, 156–159.

Grow GO (1996) Teaching learners to be self-directed. <http://www.longleaf.net/ggrow> (accessed 20 July 2005).

Hesketh EA, Laidlaw JM (2002) Developing the teaching instinct 3: facilitating learning. *Medical Teacher*, 24(5), 479–482.

†Hilton R, Morris J (2001) Student placement: is there evidence supporting team skill development in clinical practice settings? *Journal of Interprofessional Care*, 15(2), 171–183.

Hind M, Norman I, Cooper S *et al.* (2003) Interprofessional perceptions of health care students. *Journal of Interprofessional Care*, 17(1), 21–34.

†Hughes C (1999) Issues in supervisory facilitation. *Studies in Continuing Education*, 24(1), 57–71.

Hull C, Redfern L (1996) *Profiles and Portfolios*. London: Macmillan.

Ireland C (2003) Adherence to physiotherapy and quality of life for adults and adolescents with cystic fibrosis. *Physiotherapy*, 89(7), 397–407.

Johnson DW, Johnson FP (1991) *Joining Together: Group Theory and Group Skills*. Englewood Cliffs, NJ: Prentice-Hall.

Joyce B, Weil M, Showers B (1992) *Models of Teaching*. London: Allyn & Bacon.

Kitchie S (1997) Determinants of learning. In Bastable SB (ed.), *Nurse as Educator: Prinicples of Teaching and Learning*. Sudbury, MA: Jones and Bartlett Publishers.

Kolb DA (1984) *Experiential Learning*. Englewood Cliffs, NJ: Prentice-Hall.

Krathwohl DR, Bloom BS, Bertram BM (1973) *Taxonomy of Educational Objectives: The classification of educational goals, Handbook II: Affective Domain*. New York: David McKay.

†Ladyshewsky RK (2000) Peer-assisted learning in clinical education: a review of terms and learning principles. *Journal of Physical Therapy Education*, 14(2), 15–22.

Laing RD (2005) <http://www.brainyquote.com/quotes/authors/r/r_d_laing.html> (accessed 13 February 2005).

Magill MK, France RD, Munning KA (1986) Educational relationships. *Medical Teacher*, 8(2), 149–153.

Mann SJ (2005) Alienation in the learning community: a failure of community? *Studies in Higher Education*, 30(1), 43–55.

Moon JA (2000) *Reflection in Learning and Professional Development: Theory and Practice*. London: Kogan Page.

†Morris J (2003) How strong is the case for the adoption of problem-based learning in physiotherapy education in the United Kingdom? *Medical Teacher*, 25(1), 24–31.

Morrison T (2001) *Staff Supervision in Social Care*. Brighton: Pavilion Publishing.

Perry W (1970) *Forms of Intellectual and Ethical Development in the College Years*. New York: Holt, Rinehart & Winston.

Rollnick S, Mason P, Butler C (2002) *Health Behaviour Change: A Guide for Practitioners*. London: Churchill Livingstone, Chapter 2.

Roskell C, Cross V (1998) Student perceptions of cardio-respiratory physiotherapy. *Physiotherapy*, 89(1), 2–12.

Rycroft-Malone J, Kitson A, Harvey G *et al.* (2002) Ingredients for change: revisiting a conceptual framework. *Quality & Safety in Health Care*, 11(2), 174–180.

Sadlo G (1994) Problem-based learning in the development of an occupational therapy, part 2: the BSc at the London School of Occupational Therapy. *British Journal of Occupational Therapy*, 57(2), 79–84.

Schon D (1987) Educating the Reflective Practitioner. San Francisco: Jossey-Bass.

Schools of California Online Resources for Education (SCORE) (2004) Problem-based learning. <http://score.mins.k12.ca.us/problearn.html> (accessed 20 October 2004).

Scully RM, Shepard KF (1983) Clinical teaching in physical therapy education: an ethnographic study. *Physical Therapy*, 63(3), 349–358.

Soden R (1993) Vocational education for a thinking workforce – a Vygotskian perspective. *International Journal of Education and Training*, 1(1), 39–47.

Stengelhofen J (1993) *Teaching Students in Clinical Settings*. London: Chapman & Hall, Chapter 5.

**Tang S (2003) Challenge and support: the dynamics of student teachers' professional learning in the field experience. *Teaching and Teacher Education*, 19(5), 483–498.

Taras M (2002) Using assessment for learning and learning for assessment. *Assessment & Evaluation in Higher Education*, 27(6), 501–510.

Valkeavaara T (1999) 'Sailing in calm waters doesn't teach': constructing expertise through problems in work – the case of Finnish human resource developers. *Studies in Continuing Education*, 21(2), 177–196.

Waters YM, Mohanna K, Deighan M (2005) The Johari Window Model, West Midlands GP Trainers' website, Teaching resources for trainers. <http://www.trainer.org.uk/members/theory/process/johari_window.htm> (accessed 11 August 2005).

Watts NT (1990) *Handbook of Clinical Teaching: Exercises and Guidelines for Health Professionals who Teach Patients, Train Staff or Supervise Students*. London: Churchill Livingstone, Chapter 4.

*Wood BP (2000) Feedback: a key feature of medical training, *Radiology*, 215(1), 17–19.

*Wooliscroft J (2004) A suitable case for treatment? *The Clinical Teacher*, 1(1), 29–31.

Further reading

Charlin B, Mann K, Hansen P (1998) The many faces of problem-based learning: a framework for understanding and comparison. *Medical Teacher*, 20(4), 323–330.

Hayes C (2005) Clinical professional practice: a phenomenological study of teaching and learning within podiatric diabetology. *British Journal of Podiatry*, 8(2), 60–66.

*Margolis H (2005) Increasing struggling learners' self-efficacy: what tutors can do and say. *Mentoring and Tutoring*, 13(2), 221–238.

Race P, Brown S (2001) *The Lecturer's Toolkit. A Practical Guide to Learning, Teaching and Assessment*. London: Kogan Page.

Ryan SE, McKay EA (eds) (1999) *Thinking and Reasoning in Therapy*. Cheltenham: Nelson Thornes.

Whitcombe SW (2001) Using learning contracts in fieldwork education: the views of occupational therapy students and those responsible for their supervision. *British Journal of Occupational Therapy*, 64(11), 552–558.

*Wise M (2005) Using mastery learning to develop patient handling skills in occupational therapy students. *International Journal of Therapy and Rehabilitation*, 12(7), 287–293.

** Suitable for readers who wish to examine concepts at a more detailed or advanced level.
* Suitable for readers looking for something to stimulate ideas in a straightforward way.
† Included in the chapter as suggested reading.

7 ASSESSING PRACTICE-BASED LEARNING

We spend our lives assessing others, trying to know them and explain them to ourselves – and often influencing them by our subsequent decisions. (Rowntree, 1987, p. xii)

Introduction   As you have already discovered in Chapter 3, an important part of your role as a practice-based educator is to develop specific skills in practice-based assessment. The aim of this chapter is to enable you to function effectively as an assessor in the practice setting. It does this in two ways. First of all, we consider the wider educational context of practice-based assessment: the issues and perspectives that influence both the assessor's role and the assessment process itself. We ask 'What is assessment?', 'What do we assess and when?' and 'Who is involved in assessment?' Secondly, we explain the actual process of assessment. We ask 'How do we assess?' and go on to describe six steps in devising and implementing an assessment strategy.

Depending on your immediate interests, you could choose to approach this chapter in one of two ways.

- You might start at the beginning and work through each of the questions above in sequence. By doing this, you will familiarise yourself with the context of practice-based assessment, before addressing the process of developing and implementing an assessment strategy.
  OR
- You might prefer to look ahead to p. 162 and sort out the 'how to' of assessment, before going back to set this knowledge into the wider context in which practice-based assessment occurs.

PREPARATORY
REFLECTION
Working through this chapter should enable you to achieve the learning outcomes listed below. Before continuing, consider how confident you feel now in relation to them and tick the appropriate box beside each one. Are there any personal learning outcomes you would like to add to the list?

Learning outcomes

	I am confident I can do this	I am not sure I can do this
1. Define the purposes of assessment.	☐	☐
2. Identify aspects of learning that may be assessed in the practice setting.	☐	☐
3. Select from and use a range of assessment methods appropriate to the practice setting.	☐	☐
4. Describe the elements of an effective assessment strategy including validity and reliability.	☐	☐
5. Demonstrate ways in which you use assessment to facilitate others' learning and involve learners in the assessment process.	☐	☐
6. Discuss your accountability as an assessor to stakeholders in health care and education, and the implications of poor assessment practices.	☐	☐
7. Provide evidence of your own ability to learn from assessment.	☐	☐
8. Identify those aspects of the assessor role in which you feel		
○ most comfortable	☐	☐
○ least comfortable	☐	☐
○ you have a definite development need	☐	☐
and explain the reasons underlying your choice.		

Think about any personal outcomes that you would like to add to this list and make a note of them.

What is assessment?

The generally accepted meaning of 'assess' is to judge the extent of someone's learning or performance. But Freeman and Lewis (1998) point out that in education the notion of 'sitting in judgement' has only been associated with assessment since the middle of the twentieth century. A much earlier association is with the

Latin 'ad sedere', which means to sit down beside. So, in this sense, assessment is a social interaction concerned with providing guidance and feedback to learners (Brown et al., 1997). It involves identifying evidence of performance or achievement, interpreting it and taking action in response. This may generate more evidence, directly or indirectly, so that the cycle is repeated (Wiliam & Black, 1996).

The relationship between an individual learner and an individual practitioner acting as an assessor occurs in a much wider educational context. Understanding the elements of this context is important to making sense of your role as a practice-based assessor. They centre around five interrelated questions (Figure 7.1).

EXPLORATORY REFLECTION 7.1   Before continuing with the chapter, use your learning from Chapters 2–6 to make some brief notes of your initial thoughts in response to the five questions in Figure 7.1.
In what ways do you think they might be interrelated?

Why do we assess?   Based on the diagram in Chapter 3 you have probably divided the reasons for assessing into formative purposes and summative purposes. Figure 7.2 looks at these another way.

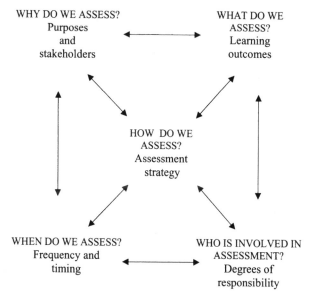

WHY DO WE ASSESS?
Purposes
and
stakeholders

WHAT DO WE
ASSESS?
Learning
outcomes

HOW DO WE
ASSESS?
Assessment
strategy

WHEN DO WE ASSESS?
Frequency and
timing

WHO IS INVOLVED IN
ASSESSMENT?
Degrees of
responsibility

Figure 7.1. The context of practice-based assessment.

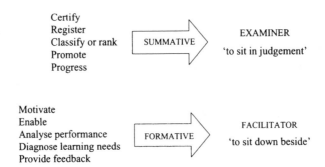

Figure 7.2. Purposes of assessment.

As we discuss later in the chapter, the distinction between these two functions can become blurred; purposes can overlap. To the extent that they generate evidence of learning and/or performance, *all* assessments could be carried out for summative reasons. But, not all assessments have an equal capacity to serve formative purposes (Wiliam & Black, 1996). However, it is possible (and desirable) to incorporate some formative features into summative assessment (Friedman Ben David, 2000).

Influence of stakeholders on assessment purposes

In Chapter 2, 'accountability' as an assessor was identified as a vital element in delivering quality health care. As a practice-based educator, your accountability extends to all those with a stake in both healthcare delivery and professional education, in particular:

- providers (employers) and consumers (patients/clients) of health care;
- providers (HEIs) and consumers (learners in the practice setting) of healthcare education;
- regulating bodies such as the Health Professions Council.

The emphasis in terms of summative and formative purposes may be seen as slightly different depending on stakeholders' perspectives. For example, Figure 7.3 illustrates how summative purposes assume greater importance from a healthcare delivery perspective, whereas formative purposes are particularly important from the perspective of learning and professional development.

Practice-based assessors are key gatekeepers of standards of service delivery, with a responsibility to safeguard the public through a robust assessment of professional competence.

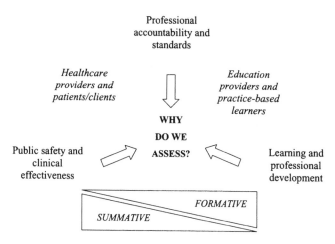

Figure 7.3. Stakeholders' influence on practice-based assessment.

A minority of incompetent professionals can do untold damage. They on their own can ultimately destroy the reputation of a profession. (Ilott and Murphy, 1999, p. 14)

Ensuring that a particular standard of performance has been achieved, which can be linked to a licence to practise, makes summative judgement the over-riding purpose in this context. Education consumers (often with a considerable financial stake in their education) have a right to expect high-quality learning experiences that will help them to develop as learners and as health professionals committed to career-long learning (Taras, 2002). This includes assessment practices that stimulate learning in a variety of ways and encourage them to learn from their mistakes. In this context, the formative function of assessment is crucial. At the same time, assessors must strive to exercise fair and accurate judgement through the use of evidence-based assessment (Tweed & Miola, 2001; Ilott & Murphy, 1999).

EXPLORATORY REFLECTION 7.2

Discuss these stakeholder perspectives with a group of colleagues.

- Who do you consider to be stakeholders in your particular situation?
- Why do you think they have an interest?

What do we assess?

From your reading in Chapter 6, you will already have realised that although an obvious answer to the question 'What do we assess?' is 'professional competence' things are not quite so simple. As you have seen, professional competence is complex

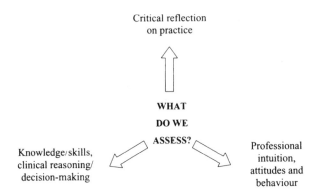

Figure 7.4. Aspects of competence encompassed by assessment.

and multifaceted, and made up of a wide variety of abilities and attributes. Developments in thinking about the relationship between learning and practice contribute to this complexity.

Figure 7.4 clusters the dimensions of professional competence into three groups. The first includes explicit (technical-rational) aspects of competence, such as acquiring theoretical knowledge and psychomotor skills, clinical reasoning and decision-making. The second includes implicit, difficult-to-demonstrate activities, such as using experience and intuition to create 'new' knowledge about practice (professional knowledge) as well as demonstrating professional attitudes and behaviour. The third includes the ability to engage in critical reflection on practice and CPD. Each of these areas is a potential focus for practice-based assessment. Learning outcomes prescribed or negotiated in relation to them must be linked directly to the assessment strategy, described below, so that learners and assessors understand clearly not only what is being assessed but also at what level.

EXPLORATORY REFLECTION 7.3

Refer back to Exploratory Reflection 6.5 in Chapter 6. Make a note of:

1. a learning outcome that focuses on a knowledge/skill-based aspect of professional competence;
2. a learning outcome associated with professional attitudes;
3. a learning outcome that reflects the ability to reflect critically on practice experience.

You will explore how these might be assessed later in this chapter.

When do we assess?

Assessment that takes place at the end of a unit of learning and is designed to act as an indicator

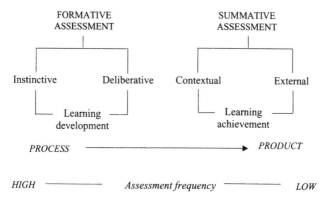

Figure 7.5. Categories and timing of assessment.

of achievement is serving a summative (or judgemental) purpose. Put another way, it is concerned with measuring a product by requiring learners to demonstrate what they know, understand or can do at a specific end point in learning (Ashcroft & Palacio, 1996). When assessment is seen as part of the ongoing learning process and learners are able to benefit immediately from feedback on their performance, then, generally speaking, its purpose is formative. However, there can be a degree of overlap between summative and formative purposes, and practice-based assessment may often have to fulfil both. In Figure 7.5, formative and summative assessments of practice-based learning are divided into categories that reflect their relative emphasis along a process–product continuum. As we explain in detail below, formative assessment may be either instinctive (occurring moment to moment) or deliberative (occurring at identified times). Summative assessment may be contextual (occurring in the practice setting) or external (occurring away from practice). Figure 7.5 also shows how formative assessment takes place more frequently than summative assessment.

Instinctive formative assessment

Teachers in the act of teaching are engaged in the process of assessing [students'] work. (Radnor & Shaw, 1995, p. 132)

. . . a teacher explaining something to an individual student may amend his or her approach almost instantaneously in response to a frown of puzzlement on the student's face or some other aspect of body language. (Wiliam & Black, 1996, p. 538)

Both of these comments demonstrate the way practice-based educators instinctively integrate the skills of formative assessment into the learning encounter without overtly disrupting the learning and teaching flow (Radnor

& Shaw, 1995). No specific assessment instruments are used; nevertheless, from moment to moment the educator builds up a substantial knowledge base about an individual learner's development by observing their reactions and by responding instinctively and spontaneously to them.

Deliberative formative assessment

This form of assessment is more explicit, with both educator and learner consciously collaborating in reviewing and developing learning. It may be initiated by the educator or the learner and involve a systematic feedback structure, such as the learning agreement described in Chapter 6.

EXPLORATORY REFLECTION 7.4

Consider the similarities between:

- instinctive formative assessment and reflection-in-action
- deliberate formative assessment and reflection-on-action
  - ○ When you engage in the instinctive and deliberate formative assessment of learners, to what extent are you also reflecting in and on your own practice as an educator?
  - ○ Discuss this in relation to some examples from your own practice

Contextual summative assessment

This category of assessment is concerned with assessing learning achievement (hence 'summative'). It is formal and structured, but still occurs within the practice context or setting. It can take a number of forms, for example:

- assessment using the negotiated criteria of the learning agreement, in a manner agreed by those involved (see Chapter 6);
- formal assessment in which the learner demonstrates her or his ability to perform specific skills or techniques on a pass/fail basis;
- assessment of overall competence by the practice-based educator based on set criteria and a rating scale.

Contextual summative assessment usually occurs at the end of a practice placement or module. It may determine progression from one stage of a programme to another or be part of a formal continuous assessment process in which students accrue grades that contribute to a final award. It may come at the end of a short practice-based course and be associated with certification.

External summative assessment

External summative assessment often draws on practice experience but takes place outside the practice setting. It may take many forms, for example:

- written or practical examinations
- essays
- seminar presentations
- projects or dissertations
- research critique.

It is beyond the immediate scope of this book, but some sources of information on summative external assessment methods are listed at the end of this chapter.

Who is involved in assessment?

Although, as we mention below, outsiders may have some input into assessment decisions, this question mainly concerns the degree of responsibility for assessment assumed by key people within the practice setting, namely educators, learners and their peers (Figure 7.6). Depicting assessment as a continuum of responsibility from unilateral, educator-controlled to learner self-assessment helps to identify these varying degrees of responsibility.

Unilateral assessment by educator

Clearly, practice-based educators have an essential part to play in any assessment of professional competence, both in terms of formative feedback for learning and in making summative judgements as gatekeepers of quality and standards. However, investing them with the sole responsibility for assessment can inhibit the achievement of many of the central goals of practice-based education.

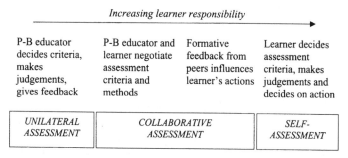

Figure 7.6. A continuum of responsibility for assessment.

EXPLORATORY
REFLECTION 7.5

Discuss some of the advantages of unilateral assessment by practice-based educators and the problems that could result from excessive reliance on this approach.

Collaborative assessment between learner and educator

One issue you may have identified in Exploratory Reflection 7.5 is that of trying to avoid anxiety on both sides about learners' readiness to take responsibility for assessment. Relinquishing or accepting responsibility can be a difficult challenge, especially for those with more traditional ideas about what students and teachers 'ought' to do (Falchikov, 1998). Collaboration is often a first step towards greater involvement of learners in the assessment process. It is exemplified by the negotiated learning agreement (see Chapter 6) in which some, or all, learning outcomes, the assessment criteria and methods are negotiated and agreed by the learner and educator together. This way assessment is more responsive to the needs and expectations of individual learners.

Collaborative peer assessment

Learners involved in the same course of study, learning alongside each other in the practice setting, are ideally placed to engage in collaborative peer assessment. However, people are often reluctant to judge their peers by awarding marks or grades; so peer assessment is used most often for formative rather than summative purposes.

Self-assessment

Successful CPD depends on the ability of individual practitioners to monitor their own performance, learn from experience and make decisions about changes in practice. Effective self-assessment is fundamental to this process. This is recognised in the broadening range of assessment tools designed to enable learners to collect, organise and interpret their own evidence of learning and achievement. We consider some of these later in the chapter. Increasing self-assessment does not mean increasing isolation from the viewpoints and opinions of others.

We see peer and self-assessing . . . as being very closely related, particularly where one is learning alongside other learners: self-assessing takes place in relation to the activities of peers, their goals, criteria, judgements, processes and products. Judgements made during self-assessing are modified by feedback from peers. (Harris & Bell, 1994, p. 113)

EXPLORATORY REFLECTION 7.6   Make a list of advantages and disadvantages of peer self-assessment from the perspective of:

1. learners
2. practice-based educators.

- Do you make use of peer assessment and/or self-assessment in your work with learners?
- What are your reasons for doing so?
- What are your reasons for not doing so?

> ... assessors must accept that putting the assessment of practice at the centre of the process brings with it increased scrutiny. As examination papers are marked by more than one teacher, then subsequently marked by external examiners, so future assessors of practice must come to accept the practice of offering a rationale for their judgements to a verifier or external examiner as part of a natural process of justice rather than ... a threatening intrusion into private mental processes.
> (Nicklin & Kenworthy, 2000, p. 115)

Role of external examiners

External examiners are appointed for professional education programmes from a list of senior educationalists compiled by the relevant professional bodies. Two or three external examiners will usually be involved with a course at any one time, being appointed for a three- to four-year period. They are primarily concerned with ensuring fairness to students and comparability of standards between similar courses elsewhere. There are a number of aspects to the external examiner's role:

- commenting on the appropriateness of assessment methods at the planning stage;
- sampling assessed work to check that decisions are consistent and appropriate;
- visiting some practice locations and discussing issues relating to a course with practitioners and learners;
- observing formal assessments at practice locations chosen at random;
- attending examination boards and assisting the programme team in making decisions about learner progression.

Thus, external examiners provide a dispassionate opinion on the quality and standards of assessment and learner performance.

At this point, you should be feeling more confident about understanding:

- what you are assessing and at what level;
- when to assess and why – when it is formative to develop learning and when it is summative to measure achievement;

- who might adopt the role of assessor and the relative advantages and disadvantages in each case.

How do we assess? Whatever the reason for assessment, the actual process involves the same basic steps (Watts, 1990):

1. choosing a focus for assessment;
2. identifying criteria to define performance;
3. setting a standard and deciding on an approach to measurement;
4. selecting a method of assessment and collecting evidence of learning and achievement;
5. interpreting the evidence and making a judgement;
6. providing feedback on assessment decisions.

These six steps comprise the assessment strategy. As a practice-based educator, you may be involved in assessment strategy at different levels. For example:

- at the level of the individual learner you may have worked through all six steps as you negotiated a learning agreement around particular elements or learning opportunities within a practice-based experience (look back to Figures 6.6 and 6.7 to remind yourself of this process);
- at the level of programme planning, as part of a combined HEI/practitioner curriculum development team; in this case, you will probably have worked through steps 1–4 to arrive at an agreed method for assessing all learners at a particular end point in, for example, an undergraduate practice-based placement or postgraduate secondment;
- at the day-to-day level you will be involved in collecting evidence of learning and achievement (step 4) to enable you (and perhaps other colleagues) to reach assessment decisions about individual learners (step 5);
- you will provide regular feedback to learners about the reasons underlying your formative and summative assessment decisions (step 6).

EXPLORATORY REFLECTION 7.7

- In your own practice situation, at what levels are you involved in assessment strategy?
- What is the nature of your particular contribution?

For an assessment strategy to be effective both in measuring achievement and stimulating learning it must link clearly to other key aspects of the learning experience, namely identified learning outcomes, design of learning experi-

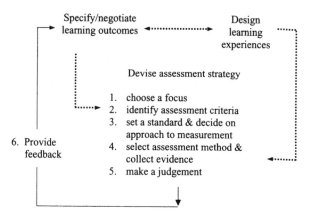

Figure 7.7. Basic steps in devising and implementing an assessment strategy.

ences and provision of feedback (Figure 7.7). If these links are not clear learners may:

- be confused and diverted from relevant learning by anxieties about summative assessment hurdles;
- fail to achieve learning outcomes because learning activities leave them inadequately prepared for assessment demands;
- not benefit from formative feedback to improve their performance.

Step 1: Choosing a focus

Choosing a focus for assessment from among the various aspects of professional competence is an important task, requiring consensus among all those involved. The focus agreed on will reflect:

- what are considered to be important priorities, for example knowledge or skill acquisition, demonstrating critical reflection skills or professional attitudes or a combination of all these;
- what learning opportunities are available, for example practitioner expertise, local availability of particular specialisms or equipment;
- the time and resources available for assessment;
- where a specific piece of assessment, such as a practice placement, fits in with the totality of assessment within a programme.

Using previously specified learning outcomes as the basis for describing the assessment focus is fundamental to effective, useful and fair assessment. They may define a generic curriculum or have been individually negotiated between learner and assessor. In either case, detailed learning outcomes go a long way towards minimising anxiety by informing learners what will be assessed and how it might be assessed. For example, a learning outcome that states:

> Learners should be able to demonstrate their ability to communicate effectively, on a day-to-day basis, with patients, carers and members of the out-patient team, using appropriate verbal and non-verbal methods

indicates that learners should expect to be observed regularly as they interact with clients and colleagues in a particular practice environment, and to have their written communications reviewed.

Step 2: Identifying assessment criteria

Although it provides useful information, the learning outcome just described says little about precisely which observable features of communication skill will actually be measured. For this, we need to decide on some assessment criteria.

> Explicit criteria help both tutors and students. They make the link between assessment and learning outcomes – they operationalise the outcomes. This helps students focus time, effort and resources on what is required. Explicit criteria make it possible for students to assess themselves and to involve others in this. (Freeman & Lewis, 1998, p. 38)

EXPLORATORY REFLECTION 7.8

In a study by Cross (2001), physiotherapy practitioners from a range of specialties identified the following as some criteria associated with effective communication in the practice setting:

1. being flexible and adaptable;
2. keeping accurate, concise and thorough records;
3. speaking clearly and audibly;
4. writing reports legibly, usefully and articulately;
5. showing interest in patients' lives and activities;
6. listening attentively with appropriate eye contact;
7. dressing professionally.

- Discuss these criteria with a group of colleagues.
- Are they what you would have expected?
- Would you want to add other criteria to the list?
- Now look at the learning outcomes you specified in Exploratory Reflection 7.3.
- Do they provide a suitable focus for assessment?

- Are they worded in such a way as to indicate clearly what is to be assessed and how it might be assessed?
- With a group of colleagues, agree on a list of appropriate assessment criteria for each outcome.

Cross (2001) Approaching consensus in clinical competence assessment. *Physiotherapy*, 87(7), 341–350.
Are you aware of any similar studies in your professional area? If so, compare the findings with those of Cross. If not, discuss the feasibility and possible outcomes of such a study in your own area of practice.

Step 3: Setting a standard and approach to measurement

Being clear about what counts as 'good' performance and what counts as 'poor' performance is what standard setting is all about. This can be approached in two different ways. First of all, in a criterion-referenced approach:

- Previously prescribed or negotiated learning outcomes linked to detailed performance criteria, such as we have described above, are used as the frame of reference.
- A level of acceptable performance or 'mastery' with which each learner's performance is compared is defined in advance.

Using a criterion-referenced standard means that all learners who have had appropriate (but not necessarily identical) learning experiences could, given sufficient time and adequate feedback, achieve all relevant criteria related to a particular learning outcome. Criterion-referenced interpretation of learning may result in:

- a dichotomous judgement that a learner has or has not mastered a particular aspect of competence (pass/fail) or
- a judgement of degree of mastery in which grades or ratings are assigned.

Rating scales used in conjunction with lists of criteria usually provide between three and seven options to quantify the level of performance above and below a minimum acceptable standard (Appendix 1 contains an example of the type of scale used). As a practice-based assessor, you have to draw on your own experience, knowledge base and clinical expertise when deciding whether the criteria have been demonstrated sufficiently for learning to be judged acceptable. Figure 7.8 summarises the relationship between the different components of criterion-referenced measurement.

The second approach to standard setting is described as 'norm-referenced'. In this approach it is not the criteria deemed to represent achievement or mastery of a particular learning outcome that define the standard but rather it

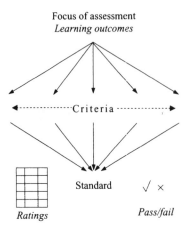

Focus of assessment
Learning outcomes

········Criteria ··········

Standard   √ ×

Ratings   *Pass/fail*

Figure 7.8. Relationship between the components of criterion-referenced measurement.

is the performance of other learners. An individual learner is assessed not in terms of pass/fail or relative mastery but in terms of 'above average', 'average' or 'below average' compared to others in her/his group. A normal distribution of scores is expected, and students at the bottom end will fail (usually with a mark of 40% or less), while those at the top end will be awarded distinctions. This approach is competitive and commonly used outside the practice setting. It enables learners' performance to be ranked, for example in university degree classification. However, although norm-referenced assessment might tell us that a learner's overall achievement is higher than that of other learners in the same group, it does not tell us whether and to what extent specific aspects of professional competence have been achieved.

EXPLORATORY
REFLECTION 7.9

A criterion-referenced approach to standard setting is not intrinsically better or worse than a norm-referenced approach. Which one is adopted depends on the purpose for which the results will be used. However, in the practice setting there are clear advantages in knowing what a learner actually knows, understands or can do, as opposed to how he or she compares with other learners.

Discuss these advantages with a group of colleagues in terms of:

• the learning process;
• your activities as a practice-based assessor;
• other stakeholders in practice-based assessment.

Step 4: Selecting an assessment method and collecting evidence

Which assessment method we choose depends, to some extent, on our purpose (summative or formative). However, in recent years the range of assessment methods used in the practice setting has expanded considerably, with emphasis being placed on assessment tasks that reflect the full variety of practice-based activity. Increasingly, methods are being used in combination so that assessment judgements are based on a holistic analysis that samples the full complexity of professional competence. The use of negotiated learning agreements is a very effective way of identifying and managing this multimethod approach. In order to gather convincing evidence, it is part of the practice-based educator's role to organise relevant learning experiences as well as assessment opportunities; ideally, the two should occur in parallel (Figure 7.7). To do this effectively, learners' current levels of knowledge and abilities must be considered, as well as learning needs and areas for development. Keeping a log of evidence can be important when you are involved with more than one learner on placement at the same time. This helps you keep track of an individual learner's progress and minimises comparisons.

Direct observation: the assessor gathers information on the learner's performance through observation and listening. Observation may take place in a one-off situation such as a clinical presentation under examination conditions. Or, evidence of learning and achievement may be accumulated gradually over time, such as the duration of a practice-based placement. In order to observe effectively you need to:

- know what you are looking for. For example, to assess performance of a psychomotor skill, you need to be able to break the task down into the component parts necessary for effective and safe execution. Is the patient positioned correctly? Is the learner positioned appropriately? Is the technique applied correctly? These points and more have to be considered when deciding what standard of performance is being demonstrated.
- where appropriate, allow sufficient time to build up an accurate impression about the standard of performance and to look for consistency at an appropriate standard. As Stoker (1994) points out, once is an event, twice is a coincidence, but three times shows that a consistent pattern is emerging.
- be aware of the possible impact of your presence on the learner and try to minimise any adverse effects ('Hawthorne' effect).

Oral/viva voce examination: this traditional face-to-face method of assessing provides a useful opportunity to assess language and interactive skills, but it can tend to focus on information recall rather than other aspects of learning. It may be useful in helping to discriminate between high-performing learners by providing challenging, in-depth questioning (Newble & Cannon, 1995). It can also be one way to assess portfolios.

Structured practical assessment: This was developed as a way of achieving a more consistent, comprehensive and efficient assessment of groups of learners in medicine (Harden, 1988), but has since been adapted and used by a variety of professions. Learners rotate around a series of stations, at which one or two aspects of competence are assessed against identical criteria using real or simulated patients. Strictly speaking, this is not a method in itself, since the range of stations can incorporate a variety of assessment methods. The aim is to assess a wide range of skills as objectively as possible.

Portfolio assessment: Unlike other methods that assess the outcomes or products of learning, portfolio assessment can be used to assess the quality of the learning processes that occurred along the way. However, this presents particular challenges for practice-based educators.

> The process that is needed does not fit neatly with the traditional concept of assessment . . . which has its roots in the science of objectivity and measurement. In order to create and, therefore, assess portfolios, we have to accept the subjectivity – almost artistic appreciation – of the work that is presented. (Snadden, Thomas & Challis, 1999, p. 9).

Challis (1999) Portfolio-based learning and assessment in medical education. *Medical Teacher*, 21(4), 370–386.

Questioning: most practice-based assessment involves questioning in some form. Phrasing questions effectively is a skill to be learnt.

- It is important to adopt an encouraging manner.
- Do not give learners the impression that you are trying to catch them out.
- The content of the question should be relevant.
- Make wording clear and precise and give learners feedback on their answers.
- Probing questions beginning with 'why' will help to reveal gaps and misconceptions.
- Bear in mind the levels of the learning taxonomies described in Boxes 6.1–6.3. Questions aimed purely at lower levels of the hierarchy will not be sufficient for assessing more advanced learners, who should be showing evidence of, for example, evaluation and synthesis of information.

EXPLORATORY REFLECTION 7.10

- Which examples of practice-based assessment methods outlined above do you consider best suited to the learning outcomes you identified in Exploratory Reflection 7.3?

- What types of learning experiences could help prepare learners to succeed in the assessments?
- Which of the methods listed have you used as an assessor or experienced as a learner?
- Are there any that you consider more suited to formative than summative purposes or vice versa?
- Are there any that you consider particularly appropriate for self-/peer assessment by learners?

Step 5: Making a judgement

Making assessment judgements is not an easy task. As a practice-based educator, you have to draw on your own experience, knowledge base and technical expertise in reaching conclusions about the standard of competence of particular learners in relation to identified criteria. However, the range of activities, assessment skills, personal attributes and environmental conditions necessary to achieve the adequate assessment of professional competence creates what Hager *et al.* (1994) describe as the 'assessment gap'.

> . . . the difference between the amount of evidence we can reasonably and reliably collect . . . and the amount of evidence which is needed to make a safe [judgement] of competence. (Hager *et al.*, 1994, p. 12).

Nevertheless, all stakeholders in professional education have a right to expect sound, evidence-based judgements from practice-based assessors. We can strive to achieve these in a number of ways.

Validity: First of all, we can ensure the validity of our assessment. In other words, does our assessment measure what we think it measures? Validity can be improved by:

- regular discussion amongst stakeholders to achieve consensus about what professional competence means in the continually changing climate of professional practice (construct validity);
- specifying learning outcomes that accord with our agreed definition of professional competence (content validity);
- using a range of relevant and appropriate assessment methods and ensuring these are carefully matched with specified learning outcomes (face validity).

Reliability: Secondly, we can improve the reliability of our assessment. In other words, how can we be sure that the same performance will be perceived in the same way by more than one assessor or by the same assessor on different assessment occasions? Reliability can be improved by:

- ensuring assessment criteria are open and transparent and their meaning commonly understood by all those involved. Often criteria are implicit and differ from assessor to assessor. Evidence from educational research shows that even where they exist, the importance attached to explicit criteria, or the extent to which evidence, personal values and assumptions contribute to decision-making, is extremely variable and not clearly understood. Regular review and discussion of assessment criteria to check for continuing consensus is essential to assure the consistency and reliability of assessment judgements.
- devising well-structured rating scales and training assessors regularly in their use, for example adhering as closely as possible to criteria and rating scales when these are available and using the full scale range. Not refusing to give certain ratings 'on principle' when they are deserved. Rating scales are only as good as the assessors who use them.
- where possible obtaining several independent ratings of the same performance.

Feasibility: Thirdly, we can make sure our assessment strategy is feasible and practicable for the context in which it is to be employed. If a particular aspect of competence cannot be accessed easily in a particular situation, it is unlikely it can be assessed adequately.

EXPLORATORY REFLECTION 7.11

Look at the example of a practice placement assessment form in Appendix 1.

- Consider what is being assessed and how the rating scale is constructed.
- With a group of colleagues, discuss the positive and negative aspects of the form.
- What do you think about the fact that it is used for both formative and summative purposes?

Warnings about assessment judgements

Unless it is possible to fail then it is unlikely that a course can guarantee professional standards. Most staff do not relish the task of conveying 'bad news', especially when a fail grade requires a student to withdraw from professional training . . . it is easy for such circumstances and consequences to interfere with the quality of decision making, especially at the margins of 'competence to practise'. (Ilott & Murphy, 1999, pp. 1–2).

At the start of this chapter, we described the assessment process as a 'social interaction' between assessors and those who are assessed. As in all such interactions, relationships and allegiances develop. Thorndike (1997) highlights an important principle in learning relationships, namely that good educators are concerned for their learners. However, this can mean that assessors are more concerned to ensure their charges get good ratings than in providing accurate information. Conversely, when relationships become disaffected, assessment judgements can be influenced adversely. It is important, as an assessor, to be self-aware – the values, attitudes and beliefs that you hold may influence your assessment judgements. It is also important to avoid bias.

Giving learners, who you know to be weak, the benefit of the doubt means:

- the learners are disadvantaged by failing to learn from their mistakes or inadequacies;
- patients may be put at risk because standards have been compromised and may continue to be compromised in the future;
- the service will acquire a weak professional;
- you have not fulfilled your professional role as a practice-based educator.

Step 6: Providing feedback

At the start of this chapter, we identified two definitions of assessment – 'to sit in judgement' (summative) and 'to sit down beside' (formative). A good assessment strategy does not simply measure achievement by requiring us to sit in judgement; it also fulfils an enabling function by asking us to sit down beside learners and provide feedback about our judgements. Earlier, we compared the involvement of practice-based educators, learners and peers in assessment. This involvement extends to the feedback component of assessment. Hence, key sources of feedback for learners include:

- educator feedback
- self-feedback
- peer feedback.

Others may also provide feedback in the practice setting, for example visiting university tutors and patients/clients.

It follows that whatever can be assessed can be the focus of feedback. Thus, practice-based assessors should be able to provide learners with a clear account of how they are progressing in relation to knowledge, psychomotor skills, critical-reflection skills, professional attitudes and behaviour.

Hesketh & Laidlaw (2002) Developing the teaching instinct 1: feedback. *Medical Teacher*, 24(3), 245–248.

EXPLORATORY REFLECTION 7.12

- Have you sought feedback on your feedback skills? If so, what have you discovered?

- Does your feedback meet the following criteria for effective feedback as described by Hesketh and Laidlaw?
  1. Avoid being judgemental. Think of feedback as 'This is what I saw – what do you think?'
  2. Give positive feedback first. This makes it easier to accept negative feedback.
  3. Focus on actions or specific examples, not vague generalisations.
  4. Avoid facial expressions and body language that convey general feedback in a non-verbal way.
  5. Don't give feedback unexpectedly. Prepare the ground, for example: 'Shall we spend a few minutes discussing . . .?'
  6. Use open questions, for example: 'How do you think that went?'
  7. If negative feedback is rejected, explore why this is. Is contrary feedback coming from elsewhere?
  8. Always make suggestions on how to remedy any learning or development needs.

Self-feedback: Enabling learners to become self-reliant in terms of feedback is an important part of learning from assessment. This means providing time and space for learners to reflect on their own practice, to observe and to appraise their own performance (using audio or video recording). Gaining confidence in their own judgement will lead them to be more proactive in eliciting feedback from you when they recognise a need. Thus, feedback becomes a collaborative rather than a one-way process. At the same time, it helps learners take on the responsibility of organising and monitoring their own CPD.

Peer feedback: Peer feedback can provide a useful means of relieving some of the pressure on busy practitioners. It also helps pre-registration and junior practitioners to understand how they are progressing in relation to their peer group, rather than in terms of qualified, experienced practitioners (Stengelhofen, 1993). It is now an accepted part of post-qualifying professional activity to be observed, appraised and at times judged by one's own professional colleagues. Facilitating peer feedback has become more important in preparing learners to accept and take on this function.

I think he [practice-based educator] got us to learn from each other quite a lot . . . so you get it from the other point of view and you are just as receptive. It's still at the same level; so it's not like you are being assessed but it's just that one of your peers is watching you and is going to help and give you some feedback at the end. (Undergraduate)

EXPLORATORY REFLECTION 7.13 Make a list of ways in which you do (or could) create opportunities for self- and peer feedback for learners in your practice setting.

Summary

This chapter has examined key issues relevant to assessment in the practice-based setting. Important points to consider are:

- Practice-based assessment is a social interaction between individuals with all that that implies.
- Stakeholders in practice-based assessment have differing expectations of the process, which assessors are required to meet.
- Practice-based assessors are important gatekeepers of professional standards.
- Whether formative or summative, practice-based assessment should be an enabling process that provides personal and professional insights, influences and improves learning and performance, enhances quality and stimulates change. In this way, the cycle of assessment is completed.

Now complete the portfolio sheet for Chapter 7.

- Check how often you are involved in the activities associated with being a practice-based assessor.
- Consider what evidence you have of your ability to fulfil ACCREDITATION OUTCOME V. Is it sufficient? If not, identify where the gaps lie and how they might be filled.
- Identify your continued development needs.
- Reassess your confidence in relation to Chapter 7's learning outcomes listed on p. 152, including any personal learning outcomes you identified for yourself.
- Complete your action plan.

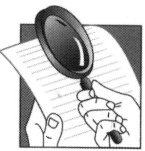

Finally, discuss the different ways in which Chapter 7 has helped you to think about your role as a practice-based assessor. What reflective purposes has the chapter served for you?

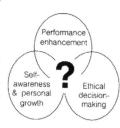

Portfolio Sheet – Assessing Practice-Based Learning

List of assessment activities	Frequency of involvement			Existing evidence for ACCREDITATION OUTCOME V (give details)	Development need?	
	Regularly	Occasionally	Never	*Apply sound principles and judgement in the assessment of performance in the clinical setting*	YES	NO
Deciding on a focus for assessment.	☐	☐	☐		☐	☐
Identifying assessment criteria.	☐	☐	☐		☐	☐
Standard setting.	☐	☐	☐		☐	☐
Selecting/devising assessment methods.	☐	☐	☐		☐	☐
Collecting evidence of learning.	☐	☐	☐		☐	☐
Making assessment judgements.	☐	☐	☐		☐	☐
Providing feedback.	☐	☐	☐		☐	☐
Instinctive formative assessment.	☐	☐	☐		☐	☐
Deliberative informative assessment.	☐	☐	☐		☐	☐
Summative contextual assessment.	☐	☐	☐		☐	☐
External summative assessment.	☐	☐	☐		☐	☐
Facilitating peer assessment and feedback.	☐	☐	☐		☐	☐
Facilitating learner self-assessment.	☐	☐	☐		☐	☐

Sufficient evidence? YES ☐ NO ☐

Chapter 7's Learning Outcomes

	I am confident I can do this	I am not sure I can do this
1. Define the purposes of assessment.	☐☐	☐☐
2. Identify aspects of learning that may be assessed in the practice setting.	☐	☐
3. Select from and use a range of assessment methods appropriate to the practice setting.	☐	☐
4. Describe the elements of an effective assessment strategy including validity and reliability.	☐	☐
5. Demonstrate ways in which you use assessment to facilitate others' learning and involve learners in the assessment process.	☐	☐
6. Discuss your accountability as an assessor to stakeholders in health care and education, and the implications of poor assessment practices.	☐	☐
7. Provide evidence of your own ability to learn from assessment.	☐	☐
8. Identify those aspects of the assessor role in which you feel	☐☐☐	☐☐☐
○ most comfortable		
○ least comfortable		
○ you have a definite development need and explain the reasons underlying your choice		

Personal learning outcomes for Chapter 7

	Confident	Not sure
	☐	☐

ACTION PLAN

Bibliography

Ashcroft K, Palacio D (1996) *Researching into Assessment and Evaluation in Colleges and Universities*. London: Kogan Page.

Brown G, Bull J, Pendlebury M (1997) *Assessing Student Learning in Higher Education*. London: Routledge.

†Challis M (1999) Portfolio-based learning and assessment in medical education. *Medical Teacher*, 21(4), 370–386.

†Cross V (2001) Approaching consensus in clinical competence assessment. *Physiotherapy*, 87(7), 341–350.

*Falchikov N (1998) Involving students in feedback and assessment. In Brown S (ed.), *Peer Assessment in Practice*. Birmingham: Staff and Educational Development Association (SEDA 102).

Freeman R, Lewis R (1998) *Planning and Implementing Assessment*. London: Kogan Page.

Friedman Ben David M (2000) The role of assessment in expanding professional horizons. *Medical Teacher*, (22)5, 472–477.

Hager H, Gonczi A, Athanasou J (1994) General issues about assessment of competence. *Assessment and Evaluation in Higher Education*, 19(1), 3–15.

Harden R (1988) What is an OSCE? *Medical Teacher*, 10(1), 19–22.

Harris D, Bell C (1994) *Evaluating and Assessing for Learning*. London: Kogan Page.

†Hesketh EA, Laidlaw JM (2002) Developing the teaching instinct 1: feedback. *Medical Teacher*, 24(3), 245–248.

**Ilott I, Murphy R (1999) *Success and Failure in Professional Education: Assessing the Evidence*. London: Whurr Publishers.

Newble D, Cannon R (1995) *A Handbook for Teachers in Universities and Colleges: A Guide to Improving Teaching Methods*. London: Kogan Page.

Nicklin PJ, Kenworthy N (eds) (2000) *Teaching and Assessing in Nursing Practice: An Experiential Approach*. London: Harcourt Publishers and the Royal College of Nursing.

Radnor H, Shaw K (1995) Developing a collaborative approach to moderation. In Torrance H (ed.), *Evaluating Authentic Assessment*. Buckingham: Open University Press.

Rowntree D (1987) *Assessing Students. How Shall We Know Them?* London: Harper & Row, Chapter 1.

Snadden D, Thomas M, Challis M (1999) *AMEE Education Guide No. 11: Portfolio-based Learning and Assessment*. Dundee: Association for Medical Education in Europe.

*Stengelhofen J (1993) *Teaching Students in Clinical Settings*. London: Chapman & Hall.

Stoker D (1994) Assessment in learning: methods of assessment. *Nursing Times*, 90(13), i–viii.

Taras M (2002) Using assessment for learning and learning from assessment. *Assessment and Evaluation in Higher Education*, 27(6), 501–510.

Thorndike RM (1997) *Measurement and Evaluation in Psychology and Education*. Englewood Cliffs, NJ: Prentice-Hall.

Tweed M, Miola J (2001) Legal vulnerability of assessment tools. *Medical Teacher*, 23(3), 312–314.

Watts NT (1990) *Handbook of Clinical Teaching: Exercises and Guidelines for Health Professionals who Teach Patients, Train Staff or Supervise Students*. London: Churchill Livingstone.

Wiliam D, Black P (1996) Meanings and consequences: a basis for distinguishing formative and summative functions of assessment? *British Educational Research Journal*, 22(5), 537–548.

Further reading

Boud D (1995) *Enhancing Learning through Self-Assessment*. London: Routledge.

Brown S (ed.) (1998) *Peer Assessment in Practice*. Birmingham: Staff and Educational Development Association (SEDA102).

*McMullan M (2005) Competence and its assessment: a review of the literature. *British Journal of Podiatry*, 8(2), 49–52.

Rust R, Wallace J (1994) *Helping Students to Learn From Each Other*. Birmingham: Staff and Educational Development Association (SEDA 86).

Welsh I, Swann C (2002) *Partners in Learning: A Guide to Support and Assessment in Nurse Education*. London: Radcliffe Medical Press.

** Suitable for readers who wish to examine concepts at a more detailed or advanced level.
* Suitable for readers looking for something to stimulate ideas in a straightforward way.
† Included in the chapter as suggested reading.

8 EVALUATING THE PRACTICE-BASED LEARNING EXPERIENCE

Introduction The reflective activities suggested in previous chapters may well have involved you in different ways of thinking about your role as a practice-based educator. They have probably led you to experiment with new or less familiar ways of acting and interacting with learners. Engaging in evaluation provides a means to explore your role further and acquire feedback on the effectiveness of your new ways of thinking and acting. As such, it is an important part of the reflective cycle. In the wider context of health care and professional education, evaluation processes are seen as increasingly important in providing evidence-based information about professional learning and its impact on service delivery. In this respect, evaluation is also perceived as a necessary activity that underpins the quality cycle.

In this chapter, we ask a great many questions. To begin with, our questions help explain what we mean by 'evaluation'. Later, we consider questions that serve as specific foci for a wide range of evaluation activities. In this respect, the chapter attempts to provide something for everyone. Depending on your role and context, you might feel parts of the chapter go beyond your immediate needs. We suggest you focus on the information and reflective activities of most use and interest to you at the moment but use the rest of the chapter to give a general sense of the wider evaluation background to practice-based learning.

PREPARATORY REFLECTION   Working through this chapter should enable you to achieve the learning outcomes listed below. Before continuing, consider how confident you feel now in relation to these outcomes and tick the appropriate box beside each one. Are there any personal outcomes you would like to add to this list?

Learning outcomes

	I am confident I can do this	I am not sure I can do this
1. Discuss the purpose(s) of evaluation and its role in enhancing the quality of practice-based learning experiences.	☐	☐
2. Develop an evaluation strategy appropriate to your needs as a practice-based educator.	☐	☐
3. Select appropriate methods for eliciting the evaluation information you require.	☐	☐
4. Analyse effectively the results of any evaluation you undertake.	☐	☐
5. Disseminate evaluation findings effectively to relevant stakeholders in the practice-based learning experience.	☐	☐
6. Use the findings of evaluations to develop and improve the quality of learning experiences for learners.	☐	☐
7. Use your involvement in the evaluation process as a tool for your own learning and professional development.	☐	☐

Think about any personal outcomes that you would like to add to this list and make a note of them.

What is evaluation and how does it differ from assessment?

In Chapter 3, we included 'evaluator' alongside 'facilitator' and 'assessor' in the multifaceted role of the practice-based educator. It is important to be clear about what we mean by 'evaluation' and 'assessment' because, internationally, these terms are quite frequently used interchangeably, causing a potential source of confusion about their purpose and conduct.

The difference simply is this: you assess your students, but you evaluate your course, your assessment of students will be part of the evaluation but only part, so the assessment tells you what and how well your students have learned. (Rowntree, 1985, p. 178)

In talking of evaluating courses [the term implies] any means by which we observe and appraise the context, the effects and the effectiveness of the teaching and learning we have set in motion. (Rowntree, 1985, p. 243)

'Assessment' focuses on learning outcomes. We use evidence of individuals' achievement in relation to such outcomes, to enable us to make judgements about what they can and cannot do as well as inferring what they might be able to do in the future. 'Evaluation', on the other hand, is the activity by which we as educators find out how successful we have been in realising our educational aims, enabling learners to fulfil their learning needs and in planning, providing and facilitating the learning experience. Evaluation is concerned with what the learning experience achieves for all the stakeholders involved, including professional and statutory bodies. This enables strategies to be developed that improve the quality of healthcare service to patients, as well as practice-placement planning, content and delivery for learners and educators. The *Practice Placement Form* in Appendix 1 and the *Practice Placement Evaluation Form* in Appendix 2 provide a useful comparison to help clarify the two terms.

EXPLORATORY REFLECTION 8.1

Think about an evaluation experience you have been involved in as a learner.

- State explicitly what was being evaluated.
- What form did the evaluation take?
- Who initiated the evaluation?
- At what stage of the learning experience did evaluation occur?
- What happened as a result of the evaluation?
- What were you told about how the evaluation information would be used?
- How did you feel about the evaluation process?

Keep your responses to hand for reference as you work through the rest of the chapter.

What does evaluation involve?

Evaluation is a rigorous procedure and, like the process of evaluating a therapeutic intervention, should be approached systematically on the basis of appropriate evidence. Therefore careful planning is essential. Coles and Grant (1985) go on to explain that evaluation is much more than just monitoring.

Many people quite legitimately have access to educational situations, observing what happens and passing comment on what they have seen, and sometimes this can lead to changes being made. But this is mere monitoring and is a somewhat amateur pursuit. An educational evaluation, however, implies judgement of merit or worth, some expression of value. The evaluator not only collects information, but also interprets, explains and makes judgements about it. Evaluators not only detect problems ... but also attempt to explain why problems have arisen and suggest remedial action ... monitoring stops at detecting the problem. (Coles & Grant, 1985, p. 3)

Anecdotal evidence that emerges during a particular learning experience may alert us initially to issues that need to be investigated. However, by undertaking systematic evaluation, educators can guard against responding precipitately to anecdotal evidence. Not only does this waste time and energy, it may actually compromise the development of the learning experience by leading us up blind alleys or diverting our attention from important issues. Although an evaluation is likely to be pre-planned, and specific methods of evaluation selected, the focus of activity can shift. In other words, it may be influenced by what is discovered along the way. With any human activity, of which learning and teaching are very complex examples, the unexpected will occur. A good evaluation strategy will allow for this unpredictability and permit it to have an appropriate influence on the process of development.

EXPLORATORY REFLECTION 8.2

Think about learning experiences you have been involved in as a provider (educator).

- How are these learning experiences evaluated?
- At what stage in the learning experience does evaluation occur?
- Who initiates the evaluation process?
- What happens to information collected during evaluation?
- What consequences have resulted from evaluation?

Keep your responses to hand for reference as you work through the rest of the chapter.

Evaluation and reflection

Like other concepts explored in this book, evaluation encompasses opposing, but at the same time complementary, ideas. It needs to be:

- systematic but flexible;
- open to subjective viewpoints but able to take an objective stance;
- looking to the future but mindful of the past;
- concerned with theory but grounded in present action.

Looked at in this way it is easy to see evaluation as a complex form of collaborative reflection on a particular educational event. Remind yourself of Kolb's (1984) cycle of reflective learning, referred to in Chapter 5 (p. 74). Kolb's cycle is systematic, but allows for movement back and forth and across the cycle. It invites subjectivity in reflective observation, but encourages objective theorising about patterns and connections between past, present and future. Finally, it requires action through experimentation with new ideas and behaviours.

In the same way that Kolb's (1984) cycle helps simplify the complexity of learning and reflection, we have created an overlapping evaluation cycle to help you visualise the interrelated elements of practice-based learning evaluation.

The overlapping cycle of evaluation

In Chapter 3, different aspects of the evaluator role were identified (see Figure 3.4). These aspects are reflected in the evaluation cycle. At the centre of the cycle is design and delivery of the practice-based learning experience. By this we mean the period of time that learners spend with you and your team in the clinical environment, and the learning activities, relationships and opportunities that occur during that time. The learning experience is linked to four key elements of the evaluation cycle: (1) identifying the purpose(s) of evaluation, (2) choosing appropriate methodologies, (3) analysing evaluation data and (4) making recommendations related to evaluation outcomes. These four elements are not necessarily sequential. They may occur concurrently, as shown by the areas of overlap in Figure 8.1. Specific implementation activities occur in these areas of overlap, namely:

- asking questions about aspects of the learning experience;
- collecting evaluation data;
- disseminating the findings of evaluation;
- planning for change or development.

These activities can recur during the cycle as they are informed by gradually emerging factors or information. Thus, the evaluation process can be dynamic and responsive, and not merely retrospective and reactive. At the same time, the cycle is systematic and, if completed rigorously, should lead to worthwhile changes and educational development.

EXPLORATORY REFLECTION 8.3

- Can you identify any similarities or parallels between the activities indicated in the evaluation cycle and those in the reflective learning cycle described in Chapter 5? Discuss this with a group of colleagues.

Developing an evaluation strategy

Anticipating evaluation is fundamental to the process of designing learning experiences, and several questions underlie any development of an evaluation strategy.

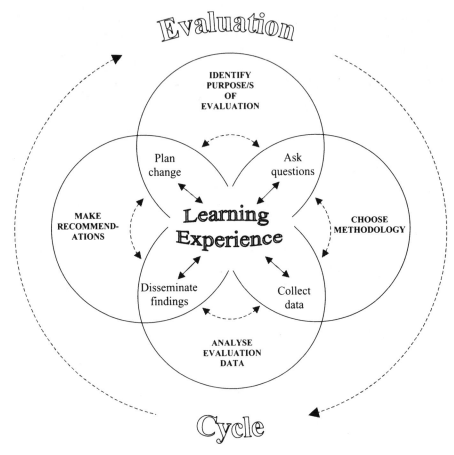

Figure 8.1. An overlapping cycle of evaluation.

1. Why do we want to evaluate, what purpose will it serve?
2. Which aspect(s) of learning experience do we want to evaluate?
3. What methodology is most appropriate for the questions we want to ask?
4. How will the data be collected and analysed?
5. When will evaluation occur?
6. Who will be involved in the process?
7. How will the data obtained through evaluation be disseminated and used to plan change?

Why do we want to evaluate?

Clearly, evaluation is not solely for the immediate participants in the learning process. It must also be acknowledged as a political activity that engages all the stakeholders mentioned earlier. Wilkes and Bligh (1999) describe three purposes of educational evaluation that have emerged over recent years. They reflect different perspectives, priorities and lines of accountability. As quality review processes focus in much more depth on practice-based learning experiences, practice-based educators are becoming involved with all three of the purposes described.

1. Participant-oriented purposes

For this purpose, those actively involved in designing and delivering the learning experience usually instigate the evaluation. This internal evaluation should help to meet the needs of both learners and practice-based educators by providing educators with feedback on their effectiveness from a range of sources and enabling them to adopt a planned approach to enhancing specific educational skills as part of their continuing professional development. Thus, internal evaluation can help you decide how you performed in terms of:

- planning (goals, content, prescribed outcomes);
- programming (delivery, resource provision, learning support);
- implementation (instigating activities, creating opportunities);
- adaptability (responding to emerging need for change or modification). (Ayers, 1989)

For learners, the result of evaluation should have a favourable impact on their personal and professional development, including their ability to achieve relevant learning outcomes.

2. Institution-oriented purposes

HEIs are concerned to uphold academic standards. As well as routine evaluation, internal audit procedures will be conducted on a regular basis. In addition, the Quality Assurance Agency (QAA) undertakes external evaluation of the quality of each institution's overall professional education provision, which includes the practice placement experience. (Refer back to Chapter 2 for an indication of the extent of QAA evaluation activity.)

3. Stakeholder-oriented purposes

Professional and statutory bodies, such as the Health Professions Council (HPC), are concerned with the development of learners into competent practitioners and members of healthcare teams, as well as with learner support and welfare systems. For example, in relation to qualifying programmes, resourcing of courses, staff–student ratios and personal tutor systems are examples of variables that are monitored regularly. In the UK, professional bodies and the HPC conduct an initial validation prior to the start of a new course programme, followed by a major review process at regular intervals as necessary. As indicated in Chapter 2, these external reviews place a strong focus on practice placements and include discussions with practice-based educators. In between revalidation events, external examiners monitor institution-based and practice-based learning as part of their ongoing role in ensuring standards are maintained.

Purchasers of education for health professionals are concerned with how well learners are prepared for current practice. They need reassurance that employers feel learners are fit for purpose. Regular educational contract reviews are conducted and clinical audit provides important information about staff efficiency and effectiveness.

If you have not done so already, now might be a good point to read the summaries of key policy documents provided in Chapter 2.

Effects of evaluation on practice-based educators

The examples of evaluation purposes outlined above help explain why educators sometimes feel threatened by the process. However open we are about submitting our work and performance for peer review, the implications of unfavourable feedback are never far from our minds!

All forms of evaluation can make you feel insecure, even threatened . . . in effect, you are submitting what you consider to be your best attempts to the scrutiny of others . . . What can be even more threatening is if these views are used for purposes which extend . . . beyond your control. (Ashcroft & Palacio, 1996, p. 119)

There is no denying the power held by purchasers who, in extreme cases, may withdraw contracts. Likewise, professional and statutory bodies can deny revalidation for professional programmes. These rare, but possible, scenarios make it vital for those concerned with practice-based learning evaluation to develop appropriate evaluation skills. This can be achieved through collaborative relationships with universities and college-based educators. Supportive practice-based learning environments that encourage and respect educators' efforts and learners' opinions also help to create an ethos of rigorous, but fair, evaluation procedures, based on constructive feedback and directed towards learning enhancement, professional development and service quality.

EXPLORATORY REFLECTION 8.4

Make a list of evaluation exercises specifically concerned with the quality of a practice-based learning experience that either you or your colleagues have been involved in.

- What was the purpose of the exercise; did it reflect any of the approaches described above?
- Who was involved?
- How was feedback conveyed to you and/or your team?
- Did any tensions arise as to how the evaluation data should be used and acted upon?
- List any possible advantages and disadvantages of internal and external evaluation in terms of
  - their objectivity;
  - perceived threat;
  - effectiveness in bringing about improvements or change.

What aspects of the learning experience do we want to evaluate?

Previous chapters have identified a wide variety of interrelated factors that could impact upon the quality and effectiveness of learning. Evaluation strategies need to take full account of this complexity. For example, it would be of limited value, at the end of a community-based placement, to use only summative assessment evidence that prescribed learning outcomes had been achieved, as a measure of placement quality. From the viewpoint of the direct participants and wider stakeholders, a multitude of factors, not reflected in such assessment evidence, may have been at work during the placement. These factors might have influenced the overall quality and longer-term impact of the experience for good or ill, for example:

- breadth and depth of clinical and social problems encountered;
- opportunities to work with a range of health- and social-care professionals in order to develop interprofessional understanding;
- levels of enthusiasm and commitment to the learning and teaching endeavour;
- number of learners attending the placement at any one time.

If we merely adopt an 'evaluation as testing' approach, by only asking how knowledgeable and skilled learners are at the end of the placement experience, there is a possibility that we will miss factors that may help us to make worthwhile improvements in areas such as:

- design of learning experiences, their content, goals and learning outcomes;
- organisation of learning experiences, including resource provision and learning support;
- addressing stakeholders' needs and expectations;
- meeting professional and educational standards.

Eliciting viewpoints for internal evaluation

Kirschling *et al.* (1995) suggest learners tend to evaluate their educators using five categories:

- use of knowledge and expertise;
- facilitative teaching methods;
- communication styles;
- use of own experience;
- giving feedback.

Feedback from one's peers is also an important source of evaluation information for the practice-based educator. Box 8.1 lists some areas in which learners are particularly well qualified to comment alongside aspects of performance on which your own peers could also be asked for useful feedback.

EXPLORATORY REFLECTION 8.5

The concept of self-evaluation is often the most neglected area of evaluation. If you have experience as a practice-based educator, do you make a point of seeking the views of learners and/or your own peers concerning your performance?

- Have you addressed any of the issues in Box 8.1?
- If so, what were the outcomes of the evaluation and how did you respond?
- If you do not seek feedback from learners and/or peers, why is this?

Box 8.1. Sources of feedback for internal evaluation
(adapted from Nelson, 1998)

Learners can provide particularly useful evaluation feedback on:
- quality of presentation of material/demonstration of skills
- the practice-based educator's teaching ability and helpfulness
- the clarity of what is taught
- degree of concern and respect for learners
- how well the practice-based educator meets learners' individual expectations
- the practice-based educator's effectiveness as a motivator of learning.

Practice-based educators' peers can provide evaluation feedback on:
- extent and currency of the practice-based educator's knowledge
- quality of the placement content
- learners' knowledge and performance
- the practice-based educator's skill and fairness in assessing learners' performance
- how well the practice-based educator meets local expectations as a practice-based educator.

- If, as yet, you have no experience as a practice-based educator, what information do you think it would be useful to find out?

Expectations of wider stakeholders

Box 8.2 contains an extract from guidelines provided by the Department of Health for England and Wales, for those in HEIs and service environments who are responsible for selecting and providing practice placements (ENB & DH, 2001). A brief summary of this document – *Placements in Focus*

Box 8.2. Guidance for education in practice for health care professions

1. Providing practice placements

1.1. Is there a jointly developed strategy agreed by HEI and service for selection, development and monitoring of practice placements?

1.2. Is the strategy for the selection and monitoring of practice placements shared with other health care education providers?

1.3. Does the strategy for the selection of practice placements enable supply to meet demand?

1.4. Is the identification of practice placements a joint exercise between HEI and service providers?

1.5. Does the strategy require a profile of practice placements?

1.6. Do all placement providers have a profile which determines:
- maximum number and type of students at any time in a placement
- the skills required by the student before beginning the practice experience
- the learning opportunities available and the learning outcomes expected from the placement?

1.7. Have practitioners working in practice areas received preparation for their role in teaching, supporting and supervising students?

1.8. Do the arrangements for practice placements enable students to have equity of opportunity for their learning experiences?

1.9. Do programme planners take account of any special needs students may have?

1.10. Does the totality of the practice experience enable the student to meet all statutory/professional requirements of the programme?

1.11. Do students and mentors/assessors know what is expected of them through specified practice outcomes?

1.12. Are placement areas designed to enable students to experience the full 24-hour a day, seven-day per week nature of health care where necessary?

1.13. Are practice placements introduced at an early stage in the programme so students can see the relevance of related theory?

1.14. Are placements of sufficient length to enable students to achieve the stated learning outcomes?

1.15. Do all students have a period of practice experience to support and consolidate their transition to registered practitioner?

1.16. Does practice experience outside the United Kingdom meet the requirements of the statutory/ professional body?

1.17. Are all placement areas audited in line with the requirements of the statutory/professional body as to their continuing suitability for students' practice experience?

1.18. Is the quality of practice placements monitored jointly by service providers and HEIs and is feedback provided to all participants?

1.19. Is good practice disseminated following audit and monitoring and does joint action planning address areas of concern or needing enhancement?

2. Practice learning environment

2.1. Does the practice area have a stated philosophy of care which is reflected in practice and supports current curriculum aims?

2.2. Does the practice provision reflect respect for the rights of health service users and their carers?

2.3. Does the provision of care reflect respect for the privacy, dignity and religious and cultural beliefs and practices of patients and clients?

2.4. Is care provision based on relevant research-based and evidence-based findings where available?

2.5. Does care provision involve different models of care commensurate with current practice and encompassing local and national initiatives?

2.6. Are interpersonal and practice skills fostered through a range of teaching/learning methods?

2.7. Does the practice experience enable students to experience the role of the registered practitioner in a range of contexts?

2.8. Do all placements have an infrastructure to support continuing professional development opportunities for practitioners?

2.9. Do students gain experience as part of a multiprofessional team?

2.10. Does the sequencing and balance between university and practice-based study promote the integration of knowledge, attitudes and skills?

2.11. Is a learning resources area available in the practice environment?

2.12. Does student feedback contribute to the ongoing evaluation of the learning environment and the student experience and are all stakeholders aware of the feedback?

3. Student support

3.1. Are students given comprehensive programme information and information about their particular placements?

3.2. Do students receive adequate and appropriate preparation for the practice placements?

3.3. Does this preparation include practice in a skills laboratory?

3.4. Do students receive a comprehensive orientation to each of their placements and is the orientation jointly agreed between mentors/assessors and programme teachers?

3.5. Are students given an initial interview during the first week of the placement, to agree the learning outcomes and ways of achieving them, taking into account their prior knowledge and experience?

3.6. Are students' learning needs, achievements and opportunities reviewed regularly?

3.7. Do students receive agreed written learning outcomes for each placement?

3.8. Do practice placements facilitate progression in terms of the learning experience available?

3.9. Does the experience available among clinical staff support the student's achievement of the learning outcomes of the educational programme at the appropriate level?

3.10. Do students receive consistent supervision and support during all practice placements?

3.11. Is there a named mentor/assessor with qualifications and experience commensurate with the context of care delivery and the requirements of the appropriate professional/statutory bodies,

3.12. who supervises and guides students in all practice placements?

3.13. Are students supported at the appropriate level in successive practice placements?

3.14. Do practice staff have dedicated time in educational activities to ensure they are competent in teaching and mentoring/assessing roles?

3.15. Do lecturers have dedicated time in practice to ensure they are competent in the practice environment?

3.16. Are lecturers involved in supporting student learning in practice areas?

3.17. Are students assisted in linking theory and practice and using a research base for practice, by lecturers and practitioners?

4. Assessment of practice

4.1. Are the periods of practice experience used for summative assessment of sufficient length to enable the agreed learning outcomes to be achieved?

4.2. Is there a named mentor/assessor with the appropriate qualifications and experience to assess students in practice placements?

4.3. Are the assessment methods used rigorous, valid and reliable?

4.4. Are there enough mentors/assessors to assess the student's developing competence and to observe the student's achievement of the intended learning outcomes over a suitable period of time?

4.5. Does the student's demonstration of competence involve the achievement of learning outcomes in both theory and practice?

4.6. Is a portfolio of practice experience included in the assessment of the student's fitness for practice?

4.7. Is the student's practice assessed in the context of a multiprofessional team?

4.8. Does the assessment strategy reflect progression, integration and coherence?

– appears in Chapter 2. The information required is categorised under four headings:

1. Providing practice placements
2. Practice learning environment
3. Student support
4. Assessment of practice

The guidelines recommend ensuring all the questions in each category are considered in planning, provision and evaluation of practice placement experiences.

EXPLORATORY   Are you surprised at the amount of information
REFLECTION 8.6   considered necessary for the evaluation of
                 practice placements?
    Consider the implications for:

• learners and educators
• higher education institutions
• service-related stakeholders

of not carrying out evaluation in each of the four categories listed.

Choosing a methodology

As with any process, one of the most important steps in carrying out an evaluation is choosing the right way to go about doing it. (Oliver & Conole, 1999)

Different methodologies represent different ideas about the process of evaluation. Which you choose depends upon what questions will provide the focus for your evaluation and what types of answers will provide the most useful information.

EXPLORATORY   Look at Question 1.7 in Box 8.2.
REFLECTION 8.7

• What additional questions might you want to ask about the practitioners' preparation for their role as educators?
• What types of answers would be most useful?

Now look at Question 3.13 in Box 8.2.

- What additional questions might you want to ask about student support during placements?
- What types of answers would be most useful?

In relation to Question 1.7 you might want to ask:

- How many practitioners receive formal preparation for their role as practice-based educators?
- How many hours' preparation is expected or required?
- How many practitioners have received professional accreditation as practice-based educators?

These questions suggest a quantitative methodology to provide data that can be used for comparative evaluation. Hence, 'yes/no' or numerical answers ('nominal' or 'interval/ratio' data, in research terminology) that can be converted to frequency tables would be most useful here.

In relation to Question 3.13 you might want to ask:

- How do learners construe 'good' support and 'poor' support?
- How does the level of support affect their enjoyment of a placement?
- What coping strategies do they employ when support seems to be inadequate for their needs?

These questions suggest a qualitative methodology to provide data that can be used for exploratory evaluation. Hence, free responses that can be used to identify influences on performance could be more useful here.

How will evaluation data be collected and analysed?

A particular feature of evaluation methodologies is the range of data we can collect. It is important that methods of data collection and their associated tools match the types of questions we want to ask.

Methods and **methodology** – what is the difference?

This is a good point at which to clarify these two terms.

By 'methods' we mean the tools and procedures used to collect evaluation data, for example using predetermined questions in a structured questionnaire or eliciting spontaneous responses in an unstructured interview. Methods are concerned with the products of evaluation.

By 'methodology' we mean the ideas and principles underlying our choice of data-collection methods. It explains why our choice of method is appropriate for the questions asked. A statement of methodology also indicates potential limitations on the generalisations or inferences we can make from our findings. Methodology is concerned with the process of evaluation.

Data-collection methods can be classified simply into listening and talking methods, observation methods, and paper and pencil techniques (Harris & Bell, 1994).

Listening and talking

Informal conversations may arise spontaneously and prove a good starting point for collecting information. They often identify areas that need more detailed investigation or guide development of the evaluation strategy.

Interviews are 'conversations with a purpose' (Robson, 1993, p. 228). They may be used for a variety of reasons (Cohen & Manion, 1990), for example:

- to discover what a person
  - knows (knowledge or information);
  - likes or dislikes (values and preferences);
  - thinks (values and beliefs);
- to help identify variables and relationships;
- to follow up unexpected findings revealed by other data-collection methods.

The type of data obtained will be determined by the interview approach. Interviews may be unstructured, semi-structured or structured, and the depth of understanding of an issue will determine the approach chosen. If little is known, an unstructured exploratory interview is appropriate. Interviewees have freedom to express their views and raise issues and concerns. Semi-structured interviews can be used when more is known about an issue. The interviewee still has scope to raise issues but the interviewer will have a guide to help maintain focus. In the structured interview, interviewees have little opportunity to raise issues of their own. Specific questions are asked in the manner of a face-to-face questionnaire.

Focus groups are organised discussions on a selected topic, within small groups of relatively homogeneous individuals. They occur in the presence of someone not directly involved with the issue(s). This person acts as a moderator, whose role is to facilitate discussion in a non-threatening, relaxed atmosphere (Thomas *et al.*, 1995).

Compared to individual interviews, which aim to obtain individual attitudes, beliefs and feelings, focus groups elicit a multiplicity of views and emotional processes within a group context. The individual interview is easier . . . to control than a focus group in which participants may take the initiative. Compared to observation, a focus group enables . . . a larger amount of information [to be gained] in a shorter period of time. (Gibbs, 1997, p. 2)

Focus groups are useful when:

- power differences exist in particular contexts;
- the prevailing culture is of interest;
- the degree of consensus on an issue needs to be explored.

Observation

> A major advantage of observation as a technique is its directness. You do not ask people about their views, feelings or attitudes; you watch what they do and listen to what they say ... This directness contrasts with, and can often usefully complement, information obtained from virtually any other technique. (Robson, 1993, p. 191)

Observation may be used as a primary method of evaluation when the purpose is to describe events or situations. It may also be used to:

- explore a situation in order to gain insights that can be tested out using other methods;
- provide supportive or supplementary evidence to complement or set existing data into perspective.

As with interviews, observation may be unstructured, which allows the unexpected to emerge and may provide rich and meaningful information, or it may be structured. Structured observation is especially useful when more open procedures have revealed an issue that is worthy of further investigation. You might also decide to invite peer observation as a source of evaluative feedback on the quality of your own performance and interaction with learners. The construction of observation guides ensures that focus is maintained and pertinent information collected. Observation may not necessarily be immediate. It may be delayed, as in the use of video recording.

Pencil and paper techniques

Assessment data, for example grades, marks, reflective accounts or professional profiles, make an important contribution to the evaluation of practice-based learning experiences. However, it goes without saying that these must be collected and used in ways that respect the anonymity and confidentiality of learners.

Self-administered questionnaires – practice placement evaluation questionnaires – are often completed by learners and educators. These tend to survey opinion on a range of factors of direct relevance to direct participants in the learning and teaching process, such as availability of resources, access to mentors, preparation of learners etc. Questions may be closed ('Did you enjoy the placement?' Yes/No), or open ('What are your feelings about the placement?'). They may involve an objective rating scale, by asking learners how far they consider prescribed learning outcomes have been achieved (0 = not at all; 7 = completely). They may incorporate a Likert scale to measure the extent of respondents' agreement or disagreement with an attitude-related statement ('I would encourage other learners to choose this placement as an option' – strongly agree/agree/disagree/strongly disagree). Questionnaires do have the advantage of collecting information relatively quickly from a large number of people. However, questionnaire design is a far more difficult task than it seems, and resulting data will only be as robust and useful as the tool used to collect it.

> A common way to end a questionnaire is to ask respondents to 'make any other comments in the space below' ... Although it may be difficult to analyze or categorize the resulting responses, these should normally be sought as a matter of principle, since they often bring out totally unexpected points or attitudes, and can add a completely new dimension to an evaluation. (Ellington & Earl, 1996, p. 3)

Data analysis

The data-collection methods we have outlined will yield a range of qualitative and quantitative data that require different approaches to analysis. For example, interview transcripts, observers' field notes and diaries, and free responses from open survey questions (qualitative data) may be interpreted through a process of coding, categorising and qualitative content analysis. Nominal, ordinal and interval/ratio data from survey questions (quantitative data) may be subjected to descriptive or inferential statistical analysis. Full details of the data-collection methods and relevant data analysis are beyond the scope of this book. However, in the further reading at the end of this chapter we draw your attention to a range of excellent texts, at a variety of levels, which will help you expand your knowledge and refine your skills in relation to those we mention and more.

Validity and reliability in evaluation

In Chapter 7, we stressed the importance of validity and reliability in relation to the design of assessment tools and the interpretation of assessment findings. The same principles apply to evaluation tools and results. Before reading on, make a note of the three definitions of validity we described in Chapter 7. If necessary, look back at p. 169 to refresh your memory.

> When choosing a method of evaluating ... it is as well to consider why we are choosing it ... How we evaluate what we are doing depends on what we think we are doing. (Raimond, 1983, p. 40)

Therefore, in the selection of evaluation methods and design of evaluation tools we must ask whether they:

- reflect consensus among stakeholders about what counts as quality in practice-based learning (construct validity);
- sample the range of stakeholder perceptions and interests adequately (content validity);
- appear relevant to the experiences of those involved in implementing the evaluation process (face validity).

We must also ask whether the methods of data collection and analysis chosen enable us to make reliable inferences from the results. Would different evaluators reach the same conclusions? Would the same evaluation on a different occasion produce similar results?

In relation to qualitative data, such as interview transcripts, observers' field notes or diaries, validity and reliability are referred to in terms of trustworthiness and rigour (Holloway & Wheeler, 1996). Here, important questions are:

- Are those contributing to the evaluation process identified and described accurately?
- Is the context in which they made their contribution explained clearly?
- Are the actions of evaluators, influences on them, and events that occurred during the data collection and analysis demonstrated clearly (is the audit trail shown)?
- Is it clear that the findings come directly from the data?

Triangulation: This involves using a range of methods in collecting data, for example observation combined with interviews (Holliday, 2002). A combination of methods that reflect both qualitative and quantitative approaches may also be used to triangulate. Triangulation creates the possibility that evidence about an evaluation issue can be confirmed from a variety of different sources. This is sometimes referred to as illuminative evaluation design because it gives scope for explanation to emerge progressively, through a process of initial examination to clarify issues, followed by further inquiry to achieve focus and direction, ending in explanation and judgement.

EXPLORATORY REFLECTION 8.8

Refer to your earlier reflections throughout this chapter.

- What data-collection methods have you encountered in your own experience of evaluation?
- Were they part of an internal or external evaluation process?

• What are your feelings about the validity and reliability or trustworthiness and rigour of the methods used and data analysis carried out?

So far, we have addressed four of our questions about evaluation, namely:

1. Why do we evaluate?
2. Which aspects of the learning experience do we want to evaluate?
3. What methodology is most appropriate?
4. How will the data be collected and analysed?

And by 'evaluation' we mean:

> ... the collection, analysis and interpretation of information about any aspect of a [learning experience], as part of a recognized process of judging its effectiveness, its efficiency and any other outcomes it may have. (Thorpe, 1988, p. 5)

Now we go on to consider the question of timing.

When does evaluation occur?

In Chapters 3 and 7, we discussed the timing of assessment in terms of summative and formative. The same concepts apply to the timing of evaluation.

Summative evaluation is carried out after a learning experience has been designed and delivered, in order to find out whether it has fulfilled its intention and objectives. Has it done the job for which it was designed, to the satisfaction of those involved and other relevant stakeholders? Summative evaluation is particularly useful for making comparisons between learning experiences, for example between iterations, types of design or delivery, or different programmes.

Formative evaluation can be carried out while a learning experience is:

• being designed or developed;
• actually taking place.

At the design/development stage, the main purpose of formative evaluation is to find out whether what is planned needs to be refined or improved in any way, and if it does can this be achieved while it is still possible to do so (Ellington & Earl, 1996)? Discussing the value of formative evaluation, Gibbs and Haigh (1983) consider why learners can seem disillusioned about evaluation exercises and why response rates to questionnaires and attendance at feedback sessions can be poor. He points out that it is usual for evaluation data, if it has any noticeable effect on learning experiences, to affect only the next iteration for the next group of learners. Very few learners actually have experience of the feedback they give improving their own situation directly. The advantage of formative evaluation is that practice-based learning experiences can be adapted as they are happening in response to ongoing feedback from learners, educators and others directly involved. As we intimated at the start of the chapter, the only cautionary note with regard to formative evaluation is the need to resist knee-jerk responses to anecdotal evidence, although this may well alert us to important issues that can be used to inform subsequent summative evaluation. The nature of formative evaluation is well illustrated in the overlapping structure of the evaluation cycle in Figure 8.1.

EXPLORATORY REFLECTION 8.9

Table 8.1 shows an overview of an illuminative evaluation design. The evaluation uses triangulation to:

1. explore the attitudes, experiences and perceptions of different groups of stakeholders in relation to the implementation of a group model of practice-based learning such as the one described in Chapter 6, p. 124;
2. find out whether the group model was a viable option and, if so, in which practice settings and circumstances it might work best;
3. ascertain the impact of the group model on the
   - quality of the learning opportunities;
   - educational and professional relationships between all those involved;
   - practice-based educators' experience of placements;
   - management of service provision in relation to the placements.

- In terms of the classification of evaluation purposes on p. 185, what would you identify as the main purpose of this evaluation?
- Is the evaluation internal or external?
- What types of questions do you think the evaluation team raised to focus the evaluation? Write some examples in the spaces provided.
- In terms of data-collection methods, which methods reflect a qualitative approach to the evaluation and which methods reflect a quantitative approach?
- In terms of timing, which elements of the evaluation are formative and which are summative?

Who is involved in evaluation?

Who initiates, designs and implements an evaluation depends largely upon the purpose of the exercise – whether this is participant-, institution- or stakeholder-oriented. But whatever the purpose, the fundamental question is 'Who is best able to provide informed feedback on the learning experience, which will assist us in making appropriate recommendations and decisions?' As we

Table 8.1. Evaluation design for a group model of practice-based learning using triangulation

PARTICIPANTS	QUESTIONS TO PROVIDE FOCUS (*Write your suggestions here*)	DATA-COLLECTION METHODS	TIMING
Practice-based educators responsible for delivering group placement experience	—	Semi-structured telephone interviews *Methodology: (tick)* ☐ *Qualitative* ☐ *Quantitative*	Prior to the practice placement ☐ *Formative* ☐ *Summative* *(tick)*
Learners attending group placements	—	Focus group discussions *Methodology: (tick)* ☐ *Qualitative* ☐ *Quantitative*	Week three of the practice placement ☐ *Formative* ☐ *Summative* *(tick)*
Practice-based educators responsible for delivering group placement experience	—	Semi-structured individual face-to-face interviews *Methodology: (tick)* ☐ *Qualitative* ☐ *Quantitative*	Immediately following the practice placement ☐ *Formative* ☐ *Summative* *(tick)*
Learners attending group placements	—	Attitude questionnaire (sent out by post) *Methodology: (tick)* ☐ *Qualitative* ☐ *Quantitative*	Dispatched two weeks after the end of the practice placement ☐ *Formative* ☐ *Summative* *(tick)*
College-based link tutors visiting learners and liaising with practice-based educators	—	Tape-recorded individual face-to-face interviews *Methodology: (tick)* ☐ *Qualitative* ☐ *Quantitative*	Immediately following the practice placement ☐ *Formative* ☐ *Summative* *(tick)*
Clinical managers covering the six pilot sites	—	Structured telephone interviews *Methodology: (tick)* ☐ *Qualitative* ☐ *Quantitative*	Two weeks after the end of the practice placement ☐ *Formative* ☐ *Summative* *(tick)*

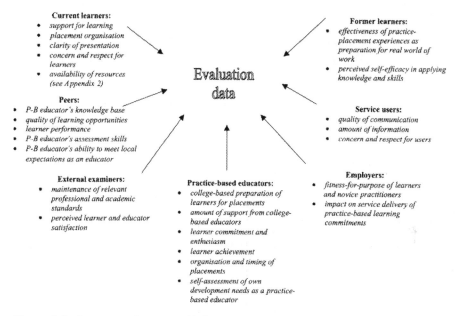

Figure 8.2. Sources and nature of informed feedback during evaluation.

have discussed above, such feedback constitutes our evaluation data and may be sought in a variety of ways, such as questionnaires, interviews, discussions etc. Some suggestions for who might be involved, and the type of feedback they could provide, are shown in Figure 8.2. You might want to add others relevant to your own particular context.

The role of learners in evaluation

Earlier in this chapter, we commented that learners were often disillusioned about evaluation and its effects. Active involvement in planning and implementing evaluation is one way to encourage greater engagement of learners with the evaluation process.

> Most course evaluation ... is designed and conducted by [educators] and rarely are students given central responsibility for planning and implementing an evaluation. Involving students as partners in educational evaluation may offer them authentic ways to develop professional skills. (Giles *et al.*, 2004, p. 681)

Now read Giles *et al.* (2004) Students as partners in evaluation: student and teacher perspectives. *Assessment and Evaluation in Higher Education*, 29(6), 681–685.

EXPLORATORY REFLECTION 8.10

- Are there any ways in which you give learners responsibility for planning and implementing aspects of the practice-based learning experience? If so, what contribution do you think it makes to their professional development?
- If you have not devolved any responsibility for evaluation to learners, discuss with colleagues some ideas to make this possible in your own context.

How will evaluation information be disseminated and used?

Dissemination is essential in the feedback link to planning change and development. Like the evaluation cycle itself, the dissemination of evaluation findings requires a systematic approach if the evidence is to be fully appreciated and understood. This is illustrated in Figure 8.3, which shows four stages of dissemination. To be effective, dissemination requires careful planning and resources, with the emphasis firmly on collaboration. A range of methods can be used, for example:

- committees, review bodies and other decision-making structures
- group discussions
- personal contacts
- workshops and in-service education events
- written reports
- websites.

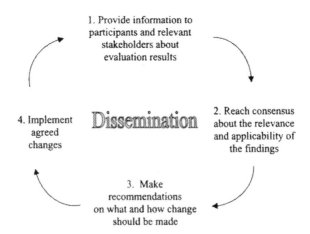

Figure 8.3. Key stages in the dissemination of evaluation findings.

EXPLORATORY REFLECTION 8.11 Look again at your reflections earlier in the chapter, on your own experiences of evaluation.

- Was evaluation information disseminated by any of the methods listed above?
- Who was present at the evaluation and what was the extent of collaboration in discussing and planning change?
- How was consensus about any change or modification achieved?
- Use the checklist below as a basis for considering the ways in which you have used the findings of any evaluation of practice-based placements offered by your department in the past.
  - ☐ Plan a personal development strategy to enhance your role as a practice-based educator.
  - ☐ Improve the quality of the placement offered in some way.
  - ☐ Influence the philosophy of the department towards practice placements.
  - ☐ Change service delivery in response to comments made by learners.
  - ☐ Make recommendations for future involvements in clinical placements.
  - ☐ Other (*give details*).

On a final note, it is worth emphasising the importance of working systematically through the evaluation cycle.

> ... before you embark on any significant piece of curriculum development that has been initiated because of evaluation feedback ... you will need to be certain that the necessity for change has been expressed strongly and *consistently*. (Ashcroft & Palacio, 1996, p. 120, original emphasis)

Armed with consistent information derived from well-designed and implemented evaluation, we can be confident of a sound evidence base for deciding on:

- aspects of the practice-based learning experience that could profitably benefit from change or further development;
- the continuing appropriateness and effectiveness of changes implemented in response to evaluation.

Summary

This chapter has examined key issues relevant to evaluating the practice-based learning experience. Important points to consider are:

- Active participation in evaluation provides valuable opportunities for learning and reflection on the practice-based educator's role.
- A systematic evaluation strategy provides a sound evidence base for change and development in practice-based education.
- There is no single best approach to evaluation. A range of methods can be used to build a comprehensive picture of the practice-based learning experience from a variety of perspectives.
- To be effective, the dissemination of evaluation findings requires a systematic process of collaboration and consensus building among all the relevant stakeholders.

Now complete the portfolio sheet for Chapter 8.

- Check how often you are involved in the activities associated with the evaluation process.
- Consider what evidence you have of your ability to fulfil ACCREDITATION OUTCOME VI. Is it sufficient? If not, identify where the gaps lie and how they might be filled.
- Identify your continued development needs.
- Reassess your confidence in relation to Chapter 8's learning outcomes listed on p. 180, including any personal learning outcomes you identified for yourself.
- Complete your action plan.

Finally, discuss the different ways in which Chapter 8 has helped you to think about your role as a practice-based assessor. What reflective purposes has the chapter served for you?

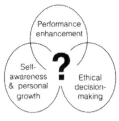

Portfolio Sheet – Evaluating the Practice-Based Learning Experience

List of evaluation activities	Frequency of involvement			Existing evidence for ACCREDITATION OUTCOME VI (give details)	Development need?	
	Regularly	Occasionally	Never	Evaluate the learning experience	YES	NO

Involvement in:
- participant-oriented evaluation
- institution-oriented evaluation
- stakeholder-oriented evaluation
- formative evaluation
- summative evaluation.

Making decisions about:
- what aspects of practice-based experiences should be evaluated;
- identifying relevant questions to provide a focus for evaluation;
- the most appropriate methodology or combination of methodologies to address evaluation questions.

Choosing appropriate methods and creating tools (e.g. questionnaires) to collect evaluation data.

Ensuring validity and reliability/trustworthiness and rigour of evaluation tools and data analysis.

Creating opportunities to evaluate your own performance as a practice-based educator by:
- soliciting peer feedback;
- inviting learners to give feedback on your performance.

Involvement in the dissemination process by:
- exchanging information;
- consensus building;
- making recommendations;
- implementing changes.

Sufficient evidence?   YES ☐   NO ☐

Chapter 8's Learning Outcomes

	I am confident I can do this	I am not sure I can do this
1. Discuss the purpose(s) of evaluation and its role in enhancing the quality of practice-based learning experiences.	☐	☐
2. Develop an evaluation strategy appropriate to your needs as a practice-based educator.	☐	☐
3. Select appropriate methods for eliciting the evaluation information you require.	☐	☐
4. Analyse effectively the results of any evaluation you undertake.	☐	☐
5. Disseminate evaluation findings effectively to relevant stakeholders in the practice-based learning experience.	☐	☐
6. Use the findings of evaluations to develop and improve the quality of learning experiences for learners.	☐	☐
7. Use your involvement in the evaluation process as a tool for your own learning and professional development.	☐	☐

Personal learning outcomes for Chapter 8

Confident	Not sure
☐	☐

ACTION PLAN

Bibliography

**Ashcroft K, Palacio D (1996) *Researching into Assessment and Evaluation in Colleges and Universities*. London: Kogan Page, Chapter 7.

Ayers JB (1989) Evaluating workshops and institutes. *Practical Assessment, Research & Evaluation*, 1(8). <http://PAREonline.net/getvn.asp?v=1&n=8> (accessed 20 February 2006).

Cohen L, Manion L (1990) *Research Methods in Education*. London: Routledge.

Coles CR, Grant JG (1985) *Curriculum Evaluation in Medical and Health Care Education*. Dundee University Centre for Medical Education: ASMEE Medical Education Research Booklet No. 1.

Ellington H, Earl S (1996) *Evaluating the Effectiveness of the Teaching/Learning Process*. Edinburgh: Napier University Centre for the Enhancement of Learning and Teaching.

English National Board for Nursing, Midwifery and Health Visiting and Department of Health (2001) Placements in focus: guidelines for education in practice for health professions, <http://www.doh.gov.uk/pdfs/places.pdf>, (accessed 27 February 2006).

Gibbs A (1997) Social research update: focus groups, <http://www.soc.surrey.ac.uk/sru/SRU19.html> (accessed 16 August 2005).

Gibbs G, Haigh M (eds) (1983) *Alternative Models of Course Evaluation Examples for Oxford Polytechnic*. SCED Occasional Paper No. 13, ISSN 0141-4183.

†Giles A, Martin SC, Bryce D, Hendry GD (2004) Students as partners in evaluation: student and teacher perspectives. *Assessment and Evaluation in Higher Education*, 29(6), 681–685.

Harris D, Bell C (1994) *Evaluating and Assessing for Learning*. London: Kogan Page.

Holliday A (2002) *Doing and Writing Qualitative Research*. London: SAGE, Chapter 4.

Holloway I, Wheeler S (1996) *Qualitative Research for Nurses*. Oxford: Blackwell Science.

Kirschling JM, Fields J, Imle M et al. (1995) Evaluating teaching effectiveness. *Journal of Nursing Education*, 34(9), 401–410.

Kolb DA (1984) *Experiential Learning*. Englewood Cliffs, NJ: Prentice-Hall.

Nelson M (1998) Peer evaluation of teaching: an approach whose time has come. *Academic Medicine*, 73(1), 4–5.

Oliver M, Conole G (1999) Learning technology dissemination initiative: evaluation cookbook, <http://www.ucbl.hw.ac.uk/ltdi/cookbook> (accessed 10 August 2005).

Raimond P (1983) Formal and informal evaluation of management courses. In Gibbs G, Haigh M (eds), *Alternative Models of Course Evaluation Examples for Oxford Polytechnic*. SCED Occasional Paper No. 13, ISSN 0141-4183.

Robson C (1993) *Real World Research: A Resource for Social Scientists and Practitioner-Researchers*. Oxford: Blackwell.

Rowntree D (1985) *Developing Courses for Students*, 2nd edn. London: Harper and Row.

Thomas L, MacMillan J, McColl E et al. (1995) Comparison of focus group and individual interview methodology in examining patient satisfaction with nursing care. *Social Sciences in Health*, 1(4), 206–220.

Thorpe M (1988) *Evaluating Open and Distance Learning.* New York: Nichols Publishing.
Wilkes M, Bligh J (1999) Evaluating educational interventions. *British Medical Journal*, 318, 1269–1272.

Further reading

Clack GB (1997) Evaluation by graduates: a tool to stimulate change? *Medical Teacher*, 19(1), 32–35.
Hicks C (2004) *Research Methods for Clinical Therapists: Applied Project Design and Analysis.* London: Churchill Livingstone.
Neary M (2000) *Teaching, Assessing and Evaluation for Clinical Competence: A Practical Guide for Practitioners and Teachers.* Cheltenham: Nelson Thornes.
*Wheeler H, Cross V, Anthony D (2000) Limitations, frustrations and opportunities: a follow-up study of nursing graduates from the University of Birmingham, England. *Journal of Advanced Nursing*, 32(4), 842–856
*Wolfhagen HAP, Gijselaers WH, Dolmans D, Essed G, Schmidt HG (1997) Improving clinical education through evaluation. *Medical Teacher*, 19(2), 99–103.

** Suitable for readers who wish to examine concepts at a more detailed or advanced level.
* Suitable for readers looking for something to stimulate ideas in a straightforward way.
† Included in the chapter as suggested reading.

9 PUTTING IT ALL TOGETHER: DEVELOPING A PRACTICE-BASED LEARNING CURRICULUM

Introduction The previous eight chapters have offered an insight into the multifaceted role of the practice-based educator and provided a toolkit of approaches and techniques that can be applied in the practice-based learning environment. This chapter is designed to help you integrate all you have learnt by working through the book. It does this using a simple model for developing a practice-placement curriculum. Put simply, a curriculum comprises all aspects of the learning and teaching experience. Here we might think of it as the ideas, concepts and skills available within a specific practice context. Thus, the model can be adapted for use with pre- or post-registration learners, patients, carers and others.

PREPARATORY REFLECTION Working through this chapter should enable you to achieve the learning outcomes listed below. Before continuing, consider how confident you feel now in relation to these outcomes and tick the appropriate box beside each one. Are there any personal learning outcomes you would like to add to this list?

Learning outcomes

	I am confident I can do this	I am not sure I can do this
1. Identify influences and constraints in your practice environment and analyse their potential impact on the learning process.	☐	☐

	I am confident I can do this	I am not sure I can do this

2. Develop a practice-based learning
   curriculum using a six-phase model that
   involves:
   ○ planning key elements of the learning
     process;
   ○ designing learning experiences and
     opportunities;
   ○ managing the learning process;
   ○ assessing achievement of learning
     outcomes;
   ○ evaluating the overall learning experience,
     including self-evaluation as a practice-
     based educator;
   ○ reflecting on the learning process and
     planning change.

Think about any personal outcomes that you would like to add to this list
and make a note of them.

**EXPLORATORY
REFLECTION 9.1**   Think about a learning experience you have
                     been involved in implementing in the past, for
                     example a placement experience for an under-
graduate or postgraduate student, or an in-service teaching session for a group
of colleagues.

• Think about any planning you undertook in preparation for the experience
  and record your thoughts for reference later.

**Developing a practice-
placement curriculum**   Figure 9.1 shows a curriculum-development
                           model we have devised to help you in the
                           planning and delivery of practice-based
learning experiences. It is made up of a central core containing a six-phase
cycle of activity:

1. Planning the learning process
2. Designing learning experiences and opportunities
3. Managing the learning process
4. Assessing learning outcomes
5. Evaluating the overall learning experience
6. Reflecting on the learning process and planning for change.

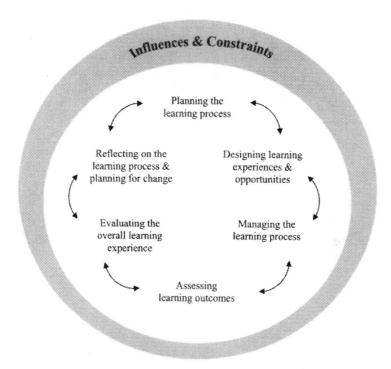

Figure 9.1. A curriculum-development model.

A ring of influences and constraints surrounds the central core, and these may affect any phase of the activity cycle.

EXPLORATORY REFLECTION 9.2

Before considering each element of the curriculum-development model, we suggest you:

- refer back to Exploratory Reflection 4.4 in Chapter 4. Choose one of the learners you listed and with whom you regularly interact. Use this learner as a basis for your reflections throughout this chapter.
- revisit the role of the practice-based educator in Chapter 3. In particular, refer back to Exploratory Reflection 3.4. What behaviours would you want to bring to the learning experiences you are planning? How do you intend to deal with, or modify, any behaviour you originally ranked at a low level?

Influences and constraints on the learning experience

A wide range of factors could influence or constrain the planning, implementation and outcomes of a learning experience. These may be environmental, attitudinal, political, managerial, psychosocial, cultural or personal in nature.

EXPLORATORY REFLECTION 9.3 Taking your own practice environment as an example, list all the influences and constraints that could affect your ability to achieve a satisfactory practice placement curriculum for your chosen learner.

The list is probably endless. You may have listed some of the following factors, along with many others:

- non-educational responsibilities in the workplace;
- amount of time available for learning and teaching activities;
- levels of learners' experience;
- organisational hierarchies and values;
- learner motivation;
- your own and colleagues' commitment to the educational programme;
- availability of resources.

Influences and constraints can be divided into those that:

- affect individual learners;
- affect the practice-based educator;
- affect the learning environment;
- reflect organisational constraints such as internal politics, financial resources and staffing levels.

Many factors may be beyond the control of learner or educator. Nevertheless, as a learning facilitator you will have to consider their potential impact on the quality and outcomes of the learning experiences you offer.

EXPLORATORY REFLECTION 9.4

- Organise your own list of influences and constraints into the four categories described above. Doing so may highlight factors you have missed.
- What do you think are the potential effects of the factors you have listed on your chosen learner, the learning experience and on you as the practice educator?
- Are there any ways in which the constraints you have identified might be modified to reduce their impact on the learning experience? Modification may not always be possible, but the exercise can help to put obstacles into perspective.

Planning the learning process As Figure 9.2 illustrates, this phase of the curriculum-development cycle involves four key activities:

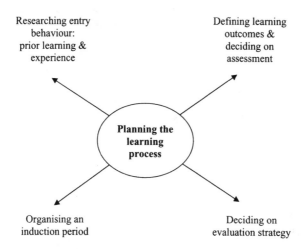

Figure 9.2. Key activities in planning the learning process.

- finding out what you can in advance about learners' prior learning and experience relevant to your placement, that is their entry behaviour;
- defining some learning outcomes in advance related to their prior learning and experience and deciding how they could be assessed – these may include prescribed or non-negotiable outcomes that apply to all learners *(Chapters 6–7)*.
- organising an induction period;
- deciding on an evaluation strategy *(Chapter 8)*.

At this stage, you may have yet to meet your learner(s). Remember, learners vary considerably in their learning needs and styles, as well as in their learning experiences. Be prepared to modify some of your plans when you eventually meet and the learners' needs become clearer, perhaps through the negotiation of a learning agreement.

Entry behaviour

'Entry behaviour' (stage of learning and life experiences of adult learners) is a term used to identify what learners bring to each new learning situation. The three learners described in Box 9.1 will have different needs and abilities. You will need to take this into account when planning learning outcomes, and when considering what facilitation methods to select from the toolkit *(Chapter 6)*.

Box 9.1. Examples of different learner entry behaviour

Learner A
- aged 20;
- A-level background in biology, statistics and psychology;
- successfully completed Year 1 of the programme;
- is about to start her first practice placement of the second year;
- diagnosed with dyslexia during first six months of the programme.

Learner B
- mature learner aged 40;
- has a BSc degree qualification in biological sciences;
- employed for 10 years as a pharmaceutical company's representative before changing career;
- now commencing his final practice-based education placement.

Learner C
- mature learner aged 30;
- employed as a healthcare assistant for four years;
- successfully completed a foundation degree as a step to entering a professional honours degree programme as a part-time student;
- has two children at primary school one of whom has a severe physical disability;
- is about to start her first practice placement.

EXPLORATORY REFLECTION 9.5

- Imagine the three learners described in Box 9.1 are pre-registration students in your profession.
- Think about the implications of their different entry behaviours for the placement-planning process.

Defining learning outcomes in advance

Usually, the learner's academic institution, in consultation with relevant practitioners in the specialty, will have identified some prescribed learning outcomes in advance. Learners receive these prior to the placement so they can prepare for the new experience by revising theoretical principles or practising specific technical skills. The practice-based educator may also define learning outcomes in advance. These often reflect local context, such as the specific experiences the placement can offer or the dynamic nature of local circumstances and constraints.

EXPLORATORY REFLECTION 9.6

- Obtain a copy of the prescribed learning outcomes for your practice area from an academic institution whose learners you support.

- Define some local learning outcomes that reflect the experience you can offer learners within the constraints you have already identified.
- If you have already defined some local learning outcomes, review these and decide whether you think they are still appropriate.

Planning how prescribed learning outcomes will be assessed

Usually, academic institutions provide a standard assessment form for pre-registration or postgraduate learners undertaking practice placements as part of their degree programme. Generally speaking, these assessment forms have been developed by a combination of academic tutors and clinical practitioners. They include a set of criteria for marking each learner's performance in areas that reflect the elements of professional competence described in Chapter 7. Assessment forms may vary between institutions, although some have adopted common tools, a development welcomed by practice-based educators supporting learners from more than one institution.

If you are planning learning experiences for other groups of learners, for example a programme of in-service education for novice practitioners or even a health-education programme for a group of patients, you will need to decide how best to assess that the learning outcomes have been met. This may involve you in designing your own customised assessment tool using the principles described in Chapter 7 and Appendix 1.

EXPLORATORY REFLECTION 9.7

- Obtain a copy of an assessment form provided by an academic institution whose learners your department supports. Analyse its content in terms of the principles described in Chapter 7, for example:
  - How are different aspects of professional competence represented or described?
  - Is the learner's performance rated or judged pass/fail?
  - Are marking criteria available?
  - Is the assessment form complemented by any other form of assessment, such as a portfolio?
  - Does it include subjective comment as well as a rating scale?
  - Does it incorporate learner feedback?
- Do you think the assessment form meets your needs and learners' needs adequately? If not, how do you think it should be modified?
- Discuss your viewpoint with academic and clinical colleagues.

Organising an induction programme

You may recognise the following extract from the Department of Health's (England and Wales) guidance for education in practice for health professionals, which we included in Chapter 8 (Box 8.2).

3.4. Do students receive a comprehensive orientation to each of their placements and is the orientation jointly agreed between mentors/assessors and programme teachers? (ENB & DH, 2001)

EXPLORATORY REFLECTION 9.8

- Have you been involved in organising induction periods for learners coming to your learning environment?
- What do you think learners need to know about the learning environment, the staff and the working practices?
- Is a period of practice observation included?
- Do you think the orientation is sufficiently comprehensive?
- Was the form and content jointly agreed between practice- and institution-based colleagues?
- Plan an induction period for a learner new to your department. Outline the activities that must take place, who will be responsible for the induction process and how long it will take.

Deciding on an evaluation strategy

As we explained in Chapter 8, evaluation is the activity by which we as educators find out how successful we have been in realising our educational aims and in enabling learners to fulfil their learning needs. Planning and design of the learning experience lie at the heart of our evaluation strategy. Although summative evaluation may occur at the end of the curriculum-development cycle, this will be influenced and informed by formative evaluation throughout the placement. Planning for evaluation means thinking about the most effective ways to find out how learners feel about you and your contribution to their learning, about the learning environment, the learning content of the placement and numerous other factors that make up the total experience.

Most academic institutions use a pro forma to elicit learners' perceptions of the quality of the learning experience as a whole. This is often dependent upon the nature of the working relationship built up between the practice-based educator and the learner. (We give an example in Appendix 2.) Think about designing your own personalised evaluation form(s) for learners and/or peers to evaluate your performance as a practice-based educator. This allows you to seek feedback on factors that are particularly important and relevant to you. For example, you might want to find out whether your questioning is sufficiently clear and a stimulus to critical reflection. You might be interested in identifying aspects of your approach that made learners feel empowered, and those they found disempowering. If your placement is optional, would learners encourage others to choose it and why?

EXPLORATORY REFLECTION 9.9

- Design an evaluation pro forma that could be used to evaluate a learning experience you have provided. Ask some colleagues to review the form to see if it is understandable and useful.
- Look back to Chapter 8 for other ways to collect evaluation information, for example listening and talking, observation and other pencil and paper techniques. Consider how and when you might use these as part of your evaluation strategy.

Designing learning experiences and opportunities This phase of the cycle involves selecting curriculum content and tailoring this to the needs of the learner.

Selecting curriculum content

In all areas of learning and teaching, curricula are finite in capacity yet have become increasingly overcrowded. Because as seasoned practitioners you are aware of and able to deal with the richness of the practice experience and the wealth of learning opportunities available, it can be easy to overestimate the capacity of learners to digest all that you can offer. There can be a tendency to try to cram them with the whole seven-course banquet, when it would be more appropriate (and humane!) to let them cut their teeth on the taster menu.

In Box 9.2 we have outlined some criteria to help in selecting curriculum content in the practice setting. When making a selection it is important to consider:

- Scope – that is, breadth and depth. This might be influenced by time constraints, the requirement for a 'common core' of experience, stage of the programme or special needs.

Box 9.2. Curriculum content selection criteria

Significance: How essential is it? Is it wholly necessary or just 'nice to know'?

Validity: How accurate or true is it? Is it evidence-based?

Applicability: How applicable is it to this particular practice context?

Appropriateness: Is the content appropriately matched to the learners' level or stage of learning?

Accessibility: Can learners gain access to the content without undue difficulty?

Interest: Does the content have intrinsic interest for the learners?

- Sequence – the order in which content is presented, for example simple to complex, pre-requisite learning or spiral sequencing in which new concepts are revisited in different contexts.

Tailoring the learning experience to individual needs

While the foregoing sections provide a good basis for drafting a curriculum and timetabling the content of the placement experience, these plans cannot be finalised until the unique perspective of the learner has been added to the design. Setting aside sufficient time during the induction period to have this introductory learning conversation is time well spent. In particular, learners' entry behaviour can be fleshed out in much more detail for the educator. In Chapter 6, we introduced a range of taxonomies (cognitive, psychomotor, affective, transferable skills) that could provide a useful basis and vocabulary for mutual exploration of where the learner is starting, in terms of knowledge, attitudes and skills acquisition. For example, inexperienced learners may have acquired factual knowledge or understanding relevant to the placement, but can they use this effectively to make reasoned clinical decisions? More-experienced or -able learners may well be able to synthesise information early on and have well-developed clinical reasoning skills, therefore how can they be challenged to progress further?

The conversation also allows the nature of local context and constraints to be made clear to the learner. For example, the learner may express a need to gain more experience of postoperative care following knee surgery. However, if few patients of this type are referred to your unit, this is a constraint that probably cannot be overcome.

As a result of your first meeting with the learner(s), you may begin to think about more appropriate methods of facilitation, or you may decide to alter the sequence of the curriculum to account for gaps in knowledge or abilities. For example, more experience in examination and assessment of simple conditions may be required before the more complex challenges you had planned can be attempted. You may decide that certain resources are now superfluous, while others may seem more essential. For example, you may need to use more X-rays in teaching than previously anticipated, or more tutorials are required than you had timetabled.

Managing the learning process

Having thoroughly planned and designed the practice-placement experience in collaboration with campus-based colleagues and the learner(s) themselves, the actual implementation should be fairly straightforward. Following induction, the learner moves into a protected clinical practice environment. You, the educator, provide that environment and help to ensure safe practice. You must decide how you facilitate the taking of responsibility, caseload-management skills, examination and assessment skills, socialisation of the learner from student to novice, or experienced to advanced practitioner etc. All these elements must be addressed in some way while also ensuring the learner experiences sufficient clinical contact. The toolkit in Chapter 6 provides a range of useful ideas. However, there are a number of important points to bear in mind.

- Remember, learning agreements, and hence the curriculum, are not completely set in stone. It may well be necessary to review some original learning outcomes. If the learner is exceptionally able or highly motivated, some planned outcomes may quickly become achieved and need to be superseded by more challenging targets or curriculum content. For other learners, early expectations may have been too high for their abilities or coping mechanisms. It may be necessary to modify some outcomes to make them more achievable or the situation less stressful, if this is inhibiting learning.
- Try to monitor the extent to which you move between the variety of roles identified in Chapter 3 and assess your effectiveness in relation to each one. Are some roles becoming more dominant than others? How does this impact upon the curriculum?
- Never underestimate the importance of feedback in helping learners improve their performance in relation to the curriculum. This means making clear decisions about how, when and where you will assess knowledge, psychomotor skills, interpersonal skills, technical abilities and the effective integration of all these (see 'Assessing learning outcomes' below). Look back to Chapters 6 and 7 to remind you of the importance and techniques of giving feedback.
- Never be afraid to tell learners the truth. If performance is poor, the learner must be told as soon as possible so that time and the opportunity to improve are not lost. Equally, learners who perform well should be openly affirmed in order to feel satisfaction and confidence in their own abilities.
- Think about developing individuals, not creating clones. Avoid trying to work to a formula.

Assessing learning outcomes

Professional competence and performance in the practice setting is commonly assessed on a continuous basis, formal feedback being given halfway through the placement period and further formal assessment taking place at the end of the placement (in Chapter 7, we referred to this as 'contextual summative assessment'). Some practice-based educators find it useful to keep an assessment log derived from all the informal feedback that occurs throughout the placement, for example following periods of observation, discussion and questioning. Collecting evidence incrementally in this way can be very helpful in informing the discussion at halfway and final assessment meetings.

As emphasised in Chapter 7, learners should also be encouraged to assess themselves prior to the formal assessment. Not only does this facilitate discussion during the formal feedback process but it also fosters CPD skills.

The results of assessment should be analysed carefully.

- Where are the weak areas?
- What can be done to help learners improve their performance?
- What specific advice can you offer the learner?

Not only does this information help current learners but it also will inform your curriculum-development planning for the next cycle of learners.

Evaluating the overall learning experience

Evaluation is crucial to curriculum development. Results from universities' student evaluation forms are sometimes fed back to practice-based educators individually. Within the institution, these are processed through the university's quality-assurance system, and, if necessary, action is taken to withdraw learners from placements that appear to be consistently unsatisfactory. As already suggested, you should feel free to evaluate any learning experience for yourself, using more of the methods you feel most comfortable with. In particular, you should make every effort to employ self- and peer evaluation of your personal contribution to curriculum development and delivery of effective and satisfying learning experiences. You may choose to keep the results private in your portfolio or you may share them with colleagues or your line manager. In any event, the information will provide a rich resource for your future curriculum-development activities and growth as a practice-based educator. Look back to Figure 8.2 to remind yourself of the range of evaluation information that could be available.

Reflecting on the learning process and planning change

It should have become clear how interdependent are the various stages of the curriculum-development cycle, for example feedback on learning could affect planning, design, management and evaluation. Thus, reflection is a continuous process throughout the cycle, making it dynamic and responsive rather than inflexible and reactive.

EXPLORATORY REFLECTION 9.10

- Using the curriculum-development model provided, draft a curriculum for a group of learners about to undertake a placement in your practice setting. Pay particular attention to how much potential for flexibility and responsiveness you are able to build in.

- Decide how you will evaluate your curriculum and, if you have the opportunity to deliver it, complete the evaluation and plan appropriate changes for the next iteration.
- If you are not yet in a position to plan a curriculum personally, find a practice educator in your environment who is, and see if you can be involved in the planning process.
- During the whole process, consider keeping a journal or making detailed notes.
- Think about how you will share your learning about the curriculum-development process with others, for example through an in-service education event or by writing a piece for a newsletter, magazine or journal.

Summary

This chapter has examined key issues relevant to developing a practice-based curriculum. Important points to consider are:

- The practice-based curriculum comprises all aspects of the learning and teaching experience including ideas, concepts and skills available within a specific practice context.
- Curriculum development is a cyclical process involving a range of interdependent activities.
- Influences and constraints associated with the practice environment may impact upon the practice-based learning process.
- Learners differ in their entry behaviour; therefore curriculum development needs to be dynamic and responsive to learners' needs as well as changing circumstances.
- Curricula are finite in capacity, therefore appropriate selection criteria should be employed to avoid overcrowding the practice-based curriculum.
- Curriculum development is a collaborative process involving practice-based educators, campus-based educators and learners.
- Evaluation is an essential part of the curriculum-development cycle.

Now complete the portfolio sheet for Chapter 9.

- Check how often you are involved in the activities associated with the curriculum-development process.
- Consider what evidence you have of your ability to pull everything together (that is integrate your learning from previous chapters) in order to fulfil ACCREDITATION OUTCOME VII. Is it sufficient? If not, identify where the gaps lie and how they might be filled.
- Identify your continued development needs.

- Reassess your confidence in relation to Chapter 9 learning outcomes listed on pp. 209–210, including any personal learning outcomes you identified for yourself.
- Complete your action plan.

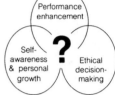

Finally, discuss the different ways in which Chapter 9 has helped you to think about your role as a practice-based assessor. What reflective purposes has the chapter served for you?

Portfolio Sheet – Developing a Practice-Based Learning Curriculum

List of curriculum-development activities	Frequency of use			Existing evidence for ACCREDITATION OUTCOME VII (give details)	Development need?	
	Regularly	Occasionally	Never		YES	NO
• Analysing the impact of environmental influences and constraints on individual learners, the practice-based educator and the learning environment.	☐	☐	☐	*Reflect on experience and formulate action plans to improve future practice*	☐	☐
• Defining some learning outcomes in advance and deciding on their assessment.	☐	☐	☐		☐	☐
• Organising an induction period.	☐ ☐	☐ ☐	☐ ☐		☐ ☐	☐ ☐
• Deciding on an evaluation strategy and designing pro formas.	☐	☐	☐		☐	☐
• Applying appropriate criteria to the selection of curriculum content, taking account of scope and sequence.	☐	☐	☐		☐	☐
• Tailoring learning experiences to individual learners' needs and entry behaviour.	☐	☐	☐		☐	☐
• Demonstrating flexibility in managing the learning experience, e.g. modifying or replacing negotiated learning outcomes.	☐	☐	☐		☐	☐
• Giving feedback and telling learners the truth.	☐ ☐	☐ ☐	☐ ☐		☐ ☐	☐ ☐
• Evaluating the practice-based learning experience to inform universities' quality assurance processes.						
• Using peer- and self-evaluation methods to inform the curriculum-development process and personal professional development.	☐	☐	☐		☐	☐
• Collaborating with campus-based colleagues and learners in curriculum development.	☐	☐	☐		☐	☐

Sufficient evidence? YES ☐ NO ☐

Chapter 9's Learning Outcomes

	I am confident I can do this	I am not sure I can do this
1. Identify influences and constraints in your practice environment and analyse their potential impact on the learning process.	☐	☐
2. Develop a practice-based learning curriculum using a six-phase model that involves:		
○ planning key elements of the learning process;	☐	☐
○ designing learning experiences and opportunities;	☐	☐
○ managing the learning process;	☐	☐
○ assessing achievement of learning outcomes;	☐	☐
○ evaluating the overall learning experience, including self-evaluation as a practice-based educator;	☐	☐
○ reflecting on the learning process and planning change.	☐	☐

Personal learning outcomes for Chapter 9

Confident	Not sure
☐	☐

ACTION PLAN

Bibliography

English National Board for Nursing, Midwifery and Health Visiting and Department of Health (2001) Placements in focus: guidelines for education in practice for health professions, <http://www.doh.gov.uk/pdfs/places.pdf> (accessed 27 February 2006).

Further reading

Keighley-James D (2002) Student participation and voices in curriculum redevelopment: the view from a curriculum development agency. *Curriculum Perspectives*, 22(1), 1–7.

APPENDIX 1

Anywhere University

SCHOOL OF HEALTHCARE PROFESSIONS

Practice Placement Assessment Form

Student Name: Practice Location:

Practice-Based Educator: Clinical Area/Specialty:

University Link Tutor:

Placement Period: From: To:

Please rate the student's performance in relation to SECTIONS A–E on a scale of 1–5 as indicated below.

1. Few criteria achieved to an   **Fail**
   acceptable standard; safety may
   have been compromised.
2. Most criteria to an acceptable   **Weak but passable performance**
   standard with some weaknesses
   that should improve experience.
3. Some criteria achieved to a high   **A good performance**
   standard; the rest are acceptable.
4. Majority of criteria achieved to a   **An excellent performance**
   very high standard.
5. All criteria achieved to an   **An outstanding performance**
   exceptionally high standard; could
   hardly be improved upon in this
   context.

A. Clinical skills and effectiveness

1. Organises own clinical workload efficiently
2. Manages time efficiently
3. Predicts likely clinical outcomes on the basis of past evidence and experience
4. Completes designated tasks fully and properly
5. Relates clinical signs and symptoms to underlying pathology
6. Works safely and effectively with patients without supervision
7. Identifies salient points of patient assessment

8. Recognises typical patterns of clinical presentation
9. Sets appropriate priorities when planning treatment
10. Selects appropriate interventions based on assessment
11. Performs interventions accurately and effectively

Rating

	Mid placement	End placement
	☐	☐

Comments

B. Patient safety & risk assessment

1. Always gives standard warnings to patients about treatments
2. Always checks for the presence of contraindications before treating patients
3. Always checks for adverse effects following treatment interventions
4. Checks relevant information before commencing treatment
5. Maintains a professional portfolio containing evidence of learning
6. Adheres to local health and safety policies
7. Checks functioning and safety of equipment used in treatment and reports faults
8. Identifies and clears hazards in environment before starting treatment
9. Asks for clinical advice or help when needed

Rating

	Mid placement	End placement
	☐	☐

Comments

C. Interpersonal skills & communication

1. Is flexible and adaptable
2. Keeps accurate, concise and thorough clinical records
3. Speaks clearly and audibly
4. Prepares reports and patient records legibly, usefully and articulately
5. Demonstrates respect for individuals' values, beliefs and practices
6. Shows appropriate interest in patients' lives and activities
7. Listens attentively and makes appropriate eye contact when assessing and treating patients
8. Dresses professionally to ensure patients' and own safety

Rating

	Mid placement	End placement
	☐	☐

Comments

D. Evidence-based practice

1. Justifies and explains own clinical decisions to peers/colleagues on the basis of research evidence
2. Accesses clinical and academic databases to inform practice
3. Rehearses new/unfamiliar techniques when appropriate opportunities arise
4. Organises time for research-related reading
5. Introduces relevant background reading into discussions about practice
6. Explains to patients why particular interventions might be desirable or inappropriate

Rating

	Mid placement	End placement
	☐	☐

Comments

E. Professional development activities & reflective practice

1. Engages in self-assessment and evaluation
2. Demonstrates treatment techniques to peers or other team members
3. Participates in and/or initiates professional dialogue within the team
4. Generates discussion with peers about aspects of learning and clinical practice
5. Tries to measure clinical outcomes for own patients
6. Tests out professional knowledge by discussing it with others
7. Selects appropriate outcome measures related to own practice
8. Is prepared to challenge existing custom and practice within the clinical environment in an informed and constructive manner
9. Demonstrates understanding of the work of other healthcare professionals and the interface between different disciplines
10. Asks for others' opinion of own work where appropriate

Rating

Mid placement	End placement
☐	☐

Comments

Enter END OF PLACEMENT ratings for Sections A–E in the chart below.

Decide the percentage mark for each section as follows:

Rating   % Mark

5 = between 70–100%
4 = between 60–69%
3 = between 50–59%
2 = between 40–49%
1 = between 0–39%

Section

	A	B	C	D	E			
Rating						Total ÷ 5		☐
% Mark						FINAL %		☐

Comments (including key strengths and weaknesses)

APPENDIX 2

Anywhere University

SCHOOL OF HEALTHCARE PROFESSIONS

Practice Placement Evaluation Form

Student Year: Practice Location:

Practice-Based Educator: Clinical Area/Specialty:

University Link Tutor:

Placement Period: From: To:

Section A

Please indicate the extent of your agreement or disagreement with EACH of the following statements related to your practice placement experience. *(Tick the appropriate box in each case)*

	Strongly agree	Agree	Disagree	Strongly disagree
1. The induction material was comprehensive and helpful	☐	☐	☐	☐
2. I felt fully integrated as part of the team	☐	☐	☐	☐
3. I was able to attend in-service education sessions	☐	☐	☐	☐
4. There was sufficient opportunity to meet other members of the team	☐	☐	☐	☐
5. Library facilities were readily available	☐	☐	☐	☐
6. I felt well prepared for the theoretical requirements of the placement	☐	☐	☐	☐
7. I felt well prepared for the practical requirements of the placement	☐	☐	☐	☐
8. I saw an appropriate selection of patients/clients	☐	☐	☐	☐

	Strongly agree	Agree	Disagree	Strongly disagree
9. My caseload was appropriate	☐	☐	☐	☐
10. I was able to achieve the core learning outcomes for the placement	☐	☐	☐	☐
11. I was able to negotiate local and personal learning outcomes	☐	☐	☐	☐
12. I was able to achieve the identified local and personal learning outcomes	☐	☐	☐	☐
13. I had regular and appropriate access to my practice-based educator	☐	☐	☐	☐
14. The practice-based educator encouraged development of relevant skills	☐	☐	☐	☐
15. The practice-based educator encouraged me to reflect on my practice and learn from my mistakes	☐	☐	☐	☐
16. The clinical educator provided positive feedback when appropriate	☐	☐	☐	☐
17. The practice-based educator provided constructive criticism when appropriate	☐	☐	☐	☐
18. I felt able to offer constructive criticism and comment about the practice experience	☐	☐	☐	☐
19. Travel information and arrangements were sufficient *(if applicable)*	☐	☐	☐	☐
20. Accommodation information and arrangements were sufficient *(if applicable)*	☐	☐	☐	☐

Section B

Add any further comments related to items 1–20 above in the space provided.
Item number:

Section C

Add any general comments or suggestions here.

Thank you for taking part in the evaluation process.

GLOSSARY

academic tutors: Tutors based in an academic institution, delivering the academic component of a programme. Their role might include visiting students whilst on placement as a link tutor (see below).

accelerated learning: Learning undertaken on an 'intensive' course in which vacation periods are shorter than normal, e.g. the content of a three-year course delivered across two years but with a similar number of weeks. Such learning requires a substantial level of commitment and an independent approach to learning from the student.

accreditation: The formal recognition of an educational programme or learning experience.

ACE Scheme: The Chartered Society of Physiotherapy's accreditation of clinical educators scheme; the CSP register recognition of the member's professional status as a practice educator via one of two routes, assessed by a higher education institution. http://www.csp.org.uk

action learning sets: A small group of people, e.g. 4–8, who meet on a regular basis to support individual members, through ongoing discussion, in identifying real workplace issues and their possible solutions. Specific action is identified and agreed by the end of each meeting, which may or may not be facilitated.

active learning: The process whereby learners actively engage in the learning process, rather than passively absorbing lectures. It involves reading, writing, discussion and engagement in solving problems, analysis, synthesis and evaluation, http://en.wikipedia.org/wiki

advanced practitioner: A (health) professional whose knowledge and skills are developed beyond those required for registration, encompassing the breadth and depth of current and likely future professional practice.

affective skills: Interpersonal and intrapersonal skills which, along with cognitive and psychomotor skills, form the basis for competence.

allied health professionals (AHPs): Members of the 13 autonomous health professions regulated by the HPC (see below), who work independently or as part of a multiprofessional healthcare team in hospitals, clinics, housing services, people's homes, schools and colleges etc., http://www.nhscareers.nhs.uk/careers/ahp/

andragogy: The art and science of helping adults learn. An approach to education in which the teacher facilitates the learner to achieve. The term is now commonly linked with theories of adult learning.

APPLE Scheme: The College of Occupational Therapists Scheme to accredit practice placement educators' professional status as practice educators via a choice of routes, assessed by a higher education institution. Adapted from the ACE Scheme, http://www.cot.org.uk/

assessment: The means by which participants' fulfilment of the aims and learning outcomes of a course are tested.

assistants: Support staff who help deliver a therapy service by working to protocols under direct or indirect supervision from qualified therapists.

autonomous learning: An approach to learning in which the learner rather than the teacher takes responsibility for goal-setting, materials selection, learning activities and assessment.

clinical supervision: A structured, formalised approach, with dedicated time for discussing professional practice with a colleague or peer that encourages reflection on, and evaluation of, clinical decision-making and outcomes.

competence: A complex synthesis of knowledge, skills, values, behaviours and attributes that enable individual professionals to work safely, effectively and legally within their particular scope of practice. Core concepts are professionalism, autonomy, self-regulation, awareness of the limits of personal practice and the practice of the profession to which individuals belong. Structured, career-long learning and development to meet identified learning needs are key elements of competence.

continuing education: Any educational activity undertaken following completion of an initial course programme.

continuing professional development (CPD): A wide range of learning activities through which professionals maintain, enhance and broaden their professional knowledge, understanding and skills throughout their careers to ensure their capacity to practise safely, effectively and legally within their evolving scope of practice is maintained.

CPD portfolio: A private resource (that might be hard copy or electronic format) that helps a professional to record, evaluate and reflect on learning and that provides a tool for identifying ongoing learning needs and planning activity to meet these. It can be used to support a range of purposes (including preparing for regular appraisal, applying for a new job, seeking academic credit for work-based learning and applying for accredited status).

cultural competence: A set of behaviours, attitudes and policies that come together as a system, agency or among professionals and enable that system, agency or those professionals to work effectively in cross-cultural situations.

distance learning: A type of education where students work on their own at home/ office and communicate with tutors and other students via a variety of forms of computer-based and other technologies.

e-learning: An approach to facilitate and enhance learning through, and based on, both computer and communications technology.

equal opportunities: An approach intended to give equal access to an environment or benefits, such as education, employment, healthcare, or social welfare to all, often with emphasis on members of various social groups which might have at some time suffered from discrimination, http://en.wikipedia.org/wiki

evaluation: An activity whereby educators endeavour to find out how successful an educational event has been in realising educational aims, enabling learners to achieve their objectives, planning, providing and facilitating learning.

evidence-based practice: An approach to healthcare in which clinicians are aware of the evidence relating to their clinical practice and are able to evaluate the strength of that evidence.

experiential learning: Learning gained through professional practice rather than through the completion of a formal course.

extended scope practitioner: A health professional working beyond the recognised scope of practice, e.g. requesting investigations, using the results of investigations to assist clinical diagnosis and appropriate management of patients; listing for surgery and referring to other medical and paramedical professionals, http://www. csp.org.uk

foundation degree: A two-year higher education qualification introduced in the UK in 2001. Aimed to give students intermediate technical and professional skills that are in demand from employers, and can give access to honours degree courses.

further education colleges: Education institutions that offer a wide range of academic, vocational, leisure and adult education courses for post-16-year-olds.

Health Professions Council (HPC): The statutory and regulatory body for the allied health professions, with protected titles. Current list (2006):

- arts therapists
- biomedical scientists
- chiropodists and podiatrists
- clinical scientists
- dieticians
- occupational therapists
- operating department practitioners
- orthoptists
- paramedics
- physiotherapists
- prosthetists and orthotists
- radiographers
- speech and language therapists.

http://www.hpc-uk.org

higher education institutions (HEIs): Institutions or universities offering qualifying and post-qualifying education.

independent learning: The learners are autonomous and responsible for their own learning.

in-service education/training: Learning in the workplace for and between health professionals. Could include a variety of activities including seminars, workshops, lectures, practical demonstrations and case discussions.

interprofessional education/learning: Situations in which professionals from two or more disciplines learn from and about each other to improve collaboration and quality of care.

learner: (in the context of this text) an undergraduate or qualified member of a healthcare profession, who is actively engaged in practice-based or work-based learning.

learner centred: A learning experience built on the needs of and driven by the learner.

learning agreement/contract: An agreement negotiated between the learner and her/his tutor which identifies the learner's specific needs together with plans for how these needs will be resourced, achieved and assessed.

learning cycle: An overlapping, cyclically phased method of learning based on action, reflection, evaluation and adjusted action.

learning outcome(s): A means of expressing learning in a way that explicitly states what learners have achieved in terms of what they know or what they can do.

learning style(s): Approach(es) to learning that reflect the individuality of the learner.

lifelong learning (LLL): The ongoing learning through which individuals maintain, enhance and broaden their knowledge, understanding and skills through formal learning opportunities and life experiences.

link tutor: A member of university staff who has responsibility for linking with the service and practice-based educator, and the learner before, during and after the placement.

module (course/programme): A self-contained component of a course/programme related to the other components; designed to offer flexibility and choice in the overall programme.

multidisciplinary team: A team of various members of the healthcare professions contribute their specific professional expertise to the identification, analysis and management of clients' problems. Their individual contributions are then coordinated as a needs related programme of intervention.

national vocational qualification (NVQ): Work-related, competence-based qualifications which reflect the skills and knowledge needed to do a job effectively and indicate that a candidate is competent in a particular area of work. No age limits or specific entry requirements.

pedagogy: The art and science of teaching children in which the teacher has full responsibility for making decisions about what will be learned, how it will be learned, when it will be learned, and if the material has been learned. The approach can be regarded as leading to dependent rather than independent, lifelong learners.

postgraduate education: Any programme of study that advances learning beyond undergraduate level.

post-registration learning/education: Any programme of study undertaken following initial professional education and state registration.

practice-based educator: An experienced work-based professional practitioner who accepts responsibility for a specific component of the clinical education programme and process.

practice education partnership: The working relationship between practice-based educator, learner, campus-based educator and clinical manager that is essential for the successful planning, organisation and conduct of the placement.

practice placements: A defined period of time, shaped by learning outcomes and assessment, within which students engage in practice-based learning to develop their knowledge, skills and understanding of the organisation and context of health-care delivery.

pre-registration learning/education: Learning associated with a programme of study that leads to the granting of a licence to practise a particular profession by the relevant statutory body.

primary care: A patient's first point of consultation.

problem-based learning: An active learning concept in which a small collaborative group of learners, with facilitation from an educator, is presented with a problem/situation as a starting point (trigger) for the identification of learning needs.

professional body: The organisation established to manage the activities of the profession.

professional registration: The qualification and/or membership process by which a person becomes recognised as a member of a specific professional body and subject to the rules of conduct and conditions of membership.

profile: Purpose-specific material, reflective statements, evidence and other material that would fit a specific use and which, on assessment, demonstrates the applicant's fulfilment of specific learning outcomes (as well as fitting within her/his broader and more private CPD portfolio).

Quality Assurance Agency (QAA): An independent body, set up in 1997, to safe-guard and enhance the quality of provision and standards of awards in the UK university structure. It is funded by subscriptions from HEIs and through contracts with HE funding bodies. QAA reviews the quality of UK HE at an institutional level, as well as academic standards and the quality of teaching and learning in each subject area (in tandem with the Department of Health, for healthcare professions, in England), http://www.qaa.ac.uk/

quality enhancement: Forward-thinking, developmental action(s)/process(es) con-cerned primarily with advising on, identifying, disseminating and promoting good practice and encouraging continuous improvement.

reflective practice: A structured process of reviewing an episode of practice to describe, analyse, evaluate and inform professional learning in such a way that new learning is identified, previous perceptions modified, understanding deepened and subsequent practice enhanced.

self-directed learning: Process by which students take responsibility for their own learning, while retaining access to advice and support from tutors.

self-efficacy: A person's perception of her/his ability to plan and take action to reach a particular goal.

tertiary care: Specialised consultative care.

work-based learning: Learning that takes place in settings that reflect the broad range of environments in which health professionals practise, that is supported, facilitated and assessed by a work/practice-based educator, and that provides opportunities for students to develop, extend, refine and consolidate learning.

INDEX